*Copyright © 2024 by Medic Mind Ltd
All rights reserved. No part of this publication may be reproduced, stored or transmitted in any form or by any means, electronic, mechanical, photocopying, recording, scanning, or otherwise without written permission from the publisher. It is illegal to copy this book, post it to a website, or distribute it by any other means without permission.*

First edition

Applying to Veterinary Medicine

Chapter 1: Deciding Where to Apply	4
Knowing the Vet School	4
Veterinary Schools	6
Bristol Veterinary School	6
Cambridge Veterinary School	8
Royal (Dick) School of Veterinary Studies (Edinburgh University)	11
Glasgow Veterinary Medicine and Surgery	13
Harper and Keele Veterinary School	15
Liverpool Institute of Veterinary Science	17
Nottingham School of Veterinary Medicine and Science	19
Royal Veterinary College London	22
Surrey School of Veterinary Medicine	25
Teaching Styles	27
Chapter 2: Work Experience	29
Work Experience Introduction	29
Small Animal Work Experience	30
Surgical Work Experience	31
Chapter 3: Applying to Veterinary Medicine	33
UCAS Veterinary Application Guide 2024	33
Chapter 4: Veterinary Personal Statement	37
Veterinary Personal Statement: The Introduction	37
Veterinary Personal Statement: Academic Interests	40
Veterinary Personal Statement: Extra-Curricular Activities	43
Veterinary Personal Statement: The Conclusion	46
Veterinary Personal Statement: Wider Reading	48
Chapter 5: The ESAT - Cambridge University Admissions Test	52
What is the ESAT?	52
ESAT Sections and Specifications	54
Top Tips for the ESAT Exam	57
Chapter 6: Veterinary Interview	59
Types of Veterinary Interview	59
What To Wear To A Vet School Interview	62
How to Prepare for a Vet School Interview	64
TOP Vet Interview Questions You Should Be Prepared To Answer	68
Veterinary Interview Scenarios & MMI Stations	72
Motivation for Veterinary Medicine	72
Work Experience	73
Personal Qualities & Skills	77
Anatomy	79

Veterinary Ethics 82
Teaching Style 83

VETERINARY LIVE MMI CIRCUIT

 Written by real MMI examiners, and trusted by schools

 Perform 10 live MMI stations yourself, completing a full circuit, and then pair up to observe an additional 10 stations!

 Experience a wide range of stations, covering role plays, veterinary ethics, hot topics, work experience, and more

Book Your Place Today!

Find out more at https://www.medicmind.co.uk/vet-school-mmi-circuit/ or scan the QR code below

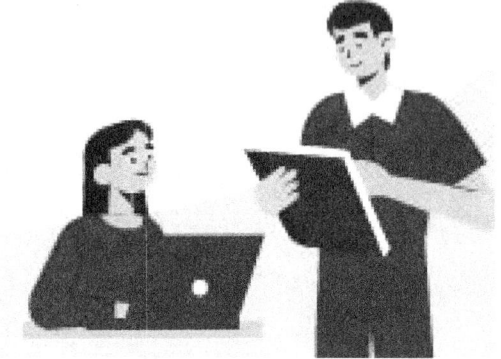

VETERINARY INTERVIEW ONLINE COURSE

 100+ tutorials, and 100+ MMI stations, designed by our Dentistry interview experts

 Learn how to answer questions on motivation for Dentistry, personal skills, work experience, hot topics, and more

 A range of packages available, including a live day of teaching and 1:1 tutoring

Buy Now!

Find out more at https://www.medicmind.co.uk/veterinary-medicine-interview-course/ or scan the QR code below

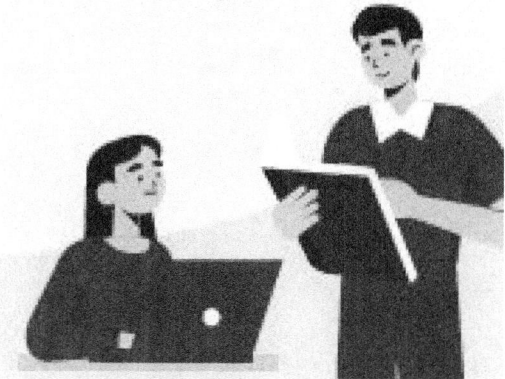

1:1 VET INTERVIEW TUTORING

 Delivered by current Dentistry students, who excelled in the interview themselves

 A personalised 1:1 approach, tailored to your unique needs

 An overall 93.4% success rate, with students improving their performance by an average of 57.3%

Book your FREE consultation now

For more information, visit https://www.medicmind.co.uk/vet-interview-tutors/ or scan the QR code below

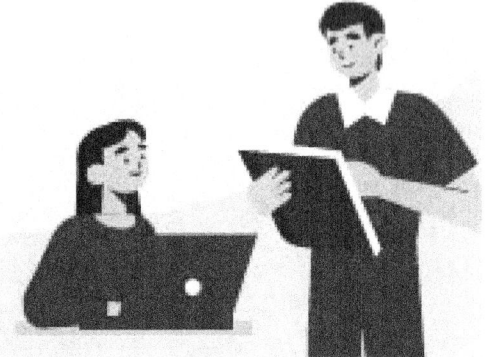

Chapter 1: Deciding Where to Apply

Knowing the Vet School
When you study veterinary medicine you are committing yourself to studying at a particular vet school for a period of several years. Universities are looking for you to have made an informed decision about not just becoming a vet but also your choice of vet school. This means you are expected to have some degree of knowledge of each vet course and the teaching that is offered.

Common Pitfall
Prospective veterinary applicants are often guided to make 'strategic applications', by applying to schools they think they are most likely to receive an offer from. Admissions panels will not see this as an acceptable reason for submitting an application. You should avoid any mention of statistics or the probability of success in your answers.

Talking about Veterinary Courses
Course structure
Research the course structure and use this to answer questions about that specific vet school. Some of the points that could be raised when discussing each vet school are listed below.

Placement locations
During your vet degree you will undertake placements at various different hospitals, farms, stables and clinics. The geographical area covered by each vet school can be quite varied and include some interesting placements. Most vet schools in the UK have two campuses, one in a city area and one in a more rural area on the outskirts of the city for farm and hospital placements. So consider how close these two campuses are to each other and make sure you like both locations.

Hospital specialisms
Some vet schools are affiliated with specialist hospitals or specialist sites . For example, students at Bristol vet school have an opportunity to visit Langfords onsite abattoir.
It is a good idea to research the vet school's main hospitals along with other facilities they have (such as equine referral units, abattoirs etc) and take note of any unique or interesting departments that tie into your own interests.

Clinical academic mix
Most vet schools require students to dedicate their first 2 years of their course to pre-clinic theory academic work which then leads onto the final 3 years based at a different campus dedicated to clinical work. Here you will be doing more animal handling. However studying veterinary medicine at Cambridge means you will dedicate 3 years to pre-clinical learning and 3 years to clinical learning.

Other opportunities
Vet school offers students a wealth of opportunities beyond acquiring a vet degree. Some universities offer the opportunity to study an intercalated degree, meaning students can obtain an additional qualification in an area of interest at BSc or Masters level. Intercalation can be compulsory or optional depending on the vet school. Intercalation allows students to direct and shape their studies according to personal interests with RVC offering a popular pathology course. If you have a particular passion or are excited to explore a specific area of veterinary medicine, mentioning this in the context of these opportunities will show you have thought about your future at that vet school.

Expert's Advice
Pay careful attention to how the vet school markets themselves. Carefully read the website or any other promotional information and take note of the key selling points that they have chosen to highlight. These points are likely the areas of the course that the vet school thinks are the most attractive. Try to incorporate these points into your answers where possible.

Veterinary Schools

Bristol Veterinary School

Overview
Bristol's modern curriculum will introduce you to the structure and function of healthy animals, the mechanisms of disease and furthermore, their clinical management. The importance of professional skills, animal health and welfare and veterinary public health are all themes which are highlighted throughout your time at Bristol and are the themes which underpin all veterinary disciplines. At Bristol vet school you will spend the first three years at the main university campus in Clifton, with at least one day a week spent at the clinical veterinary campus. The fourth and fifth years are taught purely at this separate clinical veterinary campus, with an extended, lecture-free, final clinical year.

Key points
- No interview
- Integrated BSc
- Dual campus teaching

How hard is it to get into Bristol University?
Getting into Bristol Veterinary School is highly competitive, and the application process can be challenging. The school receives a large number of applications each year, and the selection process is rigorous. However, the school does not release the acceptance rate or minimum admission requirements, so it is difficult to determine how difficult it is to get into Bristol Veterinary School. To increase your chances of being accepted, it is important to have a strong academic record, relevant work experience, and a well-written personal statement that highlights your passion for veterinary medicine.

Teaching Style
Teaching style changes across the 5 years. In the first year, you will be mostly learning via lectures, seminars etc and independent studies.

From year 1 to year 4 the amount of time in lectures and seminars decreases whilst the amount of independent studying and placement work increases.

The final 2 years are spent entirely on the Langford clinical veterinary campus where you will undergo more practical work along with your rotations in the final year - this final year is practical and clinical for the most part with minimal lectures.

University Life

In the pre-clinical years you'll be living in the university's fantastic accommodation blocks located around the centre of Bristol each with its own entertainment floor.

After these opening years you will be moving into local housing around the picturesque Langford Campus in the countryside where you will find all things veterinary such as a fantastic teaching animal hospital and a working farm.

The City of Bristol is well known for its trendy/hipster scene with a plethora of artisan cafes and vegan restaurants along with vibrant bars and clubs which will make for some unique night-life experiences. It's also a great place for sight-seeing with its hilly roads and the works of Banksy dotted around the place.

Moreover, the incredibly historic and picturesque City of Bath is only a short train journey if you're looking for a unique excursion on your days off and finally, like the other veterinary schools, Bristol university has many societies so there will probably be one for everyone.

Interview Style

If you are applying to the Gateway to Veterinary Science (Foundation programme), you will be required to attend an interview in the form of an MMI, which will take place around March. Applicants should expect to be told whether they have been successful a couple of weeks later.

Applicants may also be invited to interview if their application includes 'non-traditional' aspects. For example, if you have non-traditional qualifications or have been out of mainstream education for a long time.

Cambridge Veterinary School

Overview
The veterinary medicine department of the University of Cambridge has a world renowned reputation of prestige, excellence and world class veterinary research. If you decide to study here you can expect to go into a much higher level of detail of veterinary science and research than other universities making it the ideal choice for those with an interest in research. However if your ambition follows the more clinical route, Cambridge will still prepare you well for your career as practical sessions are common throughout the opening years and you can look forward to a final, lecture free year in which you make the most of the fantastic facilities used for rotations. Upon graduation from Cambridge Veterinary School you can expect a wider, more in-depth knowledge of veterinary science whether you go into research or into clinics.

Key points
- Veterinary science focus
- Oxbridge
- World-renowned teaching

How hard is it to get into Cambridge Veterinary School?
Getting into Cambridge Veterinary School is highly competitive and requires a strong academic background, relevant work experience, and a compelling personal statement. Admission to the school is based on a number of factors, including academic achievement, relevant work experience, and personal statement.

For the BVetMed program, applicants must have a strong academic background in science and mathematics, as well as relevant animal care experience. In addition, applicants must demonstrate excellent problem-solving and communication skills, as well as a commitment to animal welfare. The school receives a large number of applications each year and only accepts a limited number of students.

For the Veterinary Science Tripos programme, applicants must hold a degree in a related field with a minimum of a 2:1 classification. They must also demonstrate relevant work experience in veterinary science or animal care. As with the BVetMed program, competition for places is high and the school only admits a limited number of students each year.

Teaching Style
Your course at Cambridge will follow a traditional 3 years pre-clinical with the 2 final years being your clinical years.

During years 1 and 2 you will be mixed in with the medical students in order to learn the necessary core scientific knowledge. Learning will be enforced by small group teaching. Practical skills are taught from year 1, this includes 120 hours of dissection across the first 3 years. Progress is continually reviewed by your supervisors and your Director of Studies allowing the university to determine your progression through the course.

During year 4 you will undertake your Bachelor of Arts.

Years 5 and 6 consist of clinical studies. 5 involve a mixture of clinical practical sessions and lectures/small group teaching.

Your final year will be lecture free and consists entirely of practical, professional and clinical work.

University Life

The Queen's Veterinary School Hospital is only a short bus journey away from Cambridge city centre. Like many of the other veterinary schools, this campus, which consists of the majority of the necessary facilities, will be the centre of the majority of your learning. The actual surrounding area consists of a beautiful, traditional section as well as its modern counterpart.

In the old part of the city you will find a vast array of charismatic coffee shops as well as beautiful sites and architectural marvels. Along with the above, you will be living in one of the best comedic scenes in the country since Cambridge has produced some of the country's favourite comedians. Be sure to visit the annual Cambridge comedy festival as well as the 'Corn Exchange' and 'The Junction' for comedy, theatre, dance and/or other artistic performances.

Within the colleges, the social life is brilliant as well and this can be attributed to its fantastic Student Union which consists of full-time employed staff dedicated to the enjoyment and satisfaction of each and every student.

ESAT

Applicants wishing to apply to Veterinary Science at the University of Cambridge, will be required to take the ESAT (Engineering and Science Admissions Test). Please note that this has superceded this previous NSAA from 2024. For candidate applying to Veterinary Science at The University of Cambridge, the assessment comprises:

- **Mathematics 1**: All candidate (irrespective of their course choice) are required to sit this section. It consists of 27 multiple-choice questions (40 minutes)
- **Other Sections**: Candidates are also asked to sit two additional sections from the choice of: Biology, Chemistry, Physics, Mathematics 2. These sections also consist of 27 multiple-choice questions over 40 minutes.

Your performance in the assessment will not be considered in isolation, but will be taken into account alongside the other elements of your application.

For more information on the ESAT, including tips and advice, see Chapter 5 in this book.

Interview Style

Applicants that are invited to interview should expect these to take place in the first couple of weeks of December. The interviews will take the form of two panel interviews, each lasting approximately 30 minutes. Interviewers will ask a variety of questions, including your motivation to study veterinary medicine as well as some more subject-specific questions to test your aptitude in science and maths.

Royal (Dick) School of Veterinary Studies (Edinburgh University)

Overview
Edinburgh University offers a world renowned traditional/modern veterinary course hybrid. They aim to give you a variety of transferable skills such as communication, team-building and business management. This is a veterinary school that offers outstanding research-based teaching so if you are that way inclined, Edinburgh is a great veterinary school for you. Most notably, Edinburgh is widely known for its exceptional exotics department and facilities with strong links with the local Edinburgh Zoo therefore for those searching for a career in conservation or exotic clinical work Edinburgh University is a great place to start.

Key points
- Exotics
- US links
- Traditional-modern mix

Teaching Style
Years 1 and 2 consist of learning the core scientific aspects of veterinary medicine. This information is primarily communicated via lectures but wherever possible, the science will be presented in the context of its clinical relevance to give you a clear understanding of where it all leads. These opening years will also consist of sessions where you will be learning practical and clinical skills in preparation for the later years.

Years 3 to 5 will really introduce you to the clinical side of things, meaning you get an earlier introduction to this than most veterinary schools. These years consist of integrated clinical courses, each covering a different clinical area (i.e. dog and cat, farm animal etc.) Like all veterinary schools, year 5 consists of rotations.

University Life
During your time studying at the Royal (Dick) School of Veterinary Studies you'll be living in the beautiful, historical and cultured city of Edinburgh.

You can expect a friendly atmosphere created by the locals as well as a fantastic veterinary medicine centre where you will spend the majority of your course since it contains almost everything you need as a vet student.

Like Cambridge, Edinburgh has a fantastic comedic scene and is home to the famous annual 'Edinburgh Fringe' festival where you will encounter some of the country's most successful comedians as well as local and amateur comedians. This isn't the only festival in Edinburgh so you can expect a lot of special entertainment throughout the year.

In terms of night-life Edinburgh has its fair share of clubs, pubs and bars giving it a great party-scene reputation. In addition, if you're more interested in a day out you will find some great spots of culture, heritage and arts. Finally, at the actual university you'll be sure to find a suitable society or sport activity for you.

Interview Style

Interviews generally take place during December and January. Applicants that are invited to interview will be asked to take part in MMI stations. in December and January. Interview topics include:
- Motivation to study medicine and genuine interest in the medical profession
- Insight into your own strengths and weaknesses
- The ability to reflect on your own work
- Personal organisation
- Academic ability
- Problem solving
- Dealing with uncertainty
- Manage risk and deal effectively with problems Statement on the core values and attributes needed to study medicine
- Ability to take responsibility for your own actions (conscientiousness)
- Insight into your own health
- Effective communication, including reading, writing, listening and speaking
- Teamwork
- Ability to treat people with respect
- Resilience and the ability to deal with difficult situations
- Empathy and the ability to care for others
- Honesty

Glasgow Veterinary Medicine and Surgery

Overview
With over 150 years of veterinary excellence, the School of Veterinary Medicine at the University of Glasgow is pre-eminent in teaching, research and clinical provision, and attracts students, researchers and clinicians from around the world. Their research places them among the world leaders in global animal health and is top among UK veterinary schools for research quality. In essence, Glasgow's veterinary programme is designed to imbue the knowledge, philosophy, professional and technical skills such that the graduate feels confident to practice the art and science of veterinary medicine and surgery, and which prepares students for the profession that anticipates life-long learning and continuing professional development.

Key points
- 3 phase course
- Research excellence
- Spiral teaching structure

Is it hard to get into Glasgow Vet School?
Getting into Glasgow Vet School can be a highly competitive process, as the school is widely regarded as one of the best in the UK. Admission to the veterinary medicine program at Glasgow requires meeting a high academic standard, as well as demonstrating relevant work experience and a strong interest in the field.

The exact requirements for admission vary from year to year, but typically include high grades in relevant subjects such as biology and chemistry, as well as completion of relevant work experience or animal handling. Applicants are also typically required to pass an aptitude test and undergo a selection interview.

Overall, while admission to Glasgow vet school can be challenging, it is possible to gain acceptance with dedication, hard work, and a strong application. It's important to research and understand the specific requirements for admission and to seek guidance and support throughout the application process.

Teaching Style
The BVMS programme is based on integration of clinical and science subject areas and has a spiral course structure, meaning that you will revisit topics as you progress through the programme, each time with increasing clinical focus. In conjunction, there is a vertical theme of professional and clinical skills development to help you acquire the personal qualities and skills you will need in professional environments.

Through team-working and individual activities, you will develop the skills required for lifelong independent learning. The programme is delivered over five years and is divided into three phases.

Phase one (years 1 and 2) involved learning fundamental knowledge and skills.

Phase 2 (years 3 and 4) is the clinical phase. This involves the application of phase one into a clinical context.

Phase 3 is the professional phase. This is when you will gain your first hand professional veterinary experience.

University Life
The actual veterinary school is located on the outskirts of the City of Glasgow in the Garscube Campus. In the immediate surrounding area you will find its 190 hectare commercial farm along with a research centre located 5 miles to the north. Additionally, you won't be too far from Glasgow City Centre as this is located only 4 miles away.

The City of Glasgow has a brilliant and unique nightlife with more than 700 pubs and nightclubs including 100ft bars, basement clubs, converted churches and riverboats. If you're more interested in societies then you can guarantee you will find the right one for you with its 200+ clubs and societies distributed across its campuses. On the actual Garscube Campus, which is where you will spend the majority of your time during this course you will find exceptional indoor and outdoor facilities.

Interview Style
Successful applicants will be invited to interview between December and February. There will be two panel interviews, each of approximately 15 minutes. There will also be a computer-based exercise that tests applicant's understanding of ethical awareness and critical thinking skills. Common interview topics include:
- Hobbies and interests
- School work
- Knowledge of the veterinary profession
- An understanding of the realities of the veterinary world
- Personal attributes
- Current affairs

Harper and Keele Veterinary School

Overview
Harper and Keele is a brand new veterinary school that is brought to you by joint effort of Keele University, which has been offering a medicine course for a while now, and Harper-Adams, a university specialising in animal and agricultural sciences. With their combined knowledge and expertise they aim to bring you a novel veterinary course that will make the most of the facilities and experience of each campus. Like Surrey and Nottingham Veterinary Schools, Harper-Keele will promote a practical hands-on approach to learning along with an emphasis on case-based learning. You can also expect a lot of weight to be placed on large animal veterinary along with a large variety of on-campus animals from your average house-hold pet to nocturnal species.

Key points
- 2 campuses
- Farm on campus
- Companion animal facilities

Teaching Style
As aforementioned, this is a highly practical course. They will also integrate a clinical context from year 1. In order to facilitate this learning style the following methods are used: Exposure to the farm and companion animals on site at Harper Adams along with the laboratory facilities found at both Harper and Keele are maximised – you will spend a lot of time around these.

Small group teaching to facilitate information from lectures and develop the confidence of individual students. Case study based learning is used to integrate a real life clinical context into the teaching. Clinical teaching offers a variety of cases.

Lectures are led by experienced educators and practical classes/tutorials will make use of practising vets and clinical specialists to deliver the lessons.

University Life
Harper Adams – Shropshire
This small homely campus is located in the heart of the beautiful Shropshire countryside. You will find a variety of animal handling facilities as well as a teaching hospital on this campus as well as an on-campus farm.

Keele – Staffordshire
As the larger of the two campuses, Keele offers a more authentic campus experience. You can expect fantastic teaching facilities and laboratories as well as a vibrant on-campus club but the trade-off is the lack of handling facilities on campus.

Since the surrounding area is fairly quiet you can find almost everything you need on-campus. Both campuses have on-site clubs/pubs to satisfy your night-life as well as local pubs in the area. The student-union is quite pro-active in organising fun events for the students so you can expect to be entertained on your nights out. Each campus has a large range of clubs and societies as well as their own sports-centres. The greatest advantage of Harper-Keele in terms of social life is the opportunity to make the most of events, facilities and societies of both campuses meaning if you can't find what you need on one, the chances are you'll find it on the other.

Interview Style
If successful, applicants will be invited to take part in MMI stations between November and March. Interview topics include:
- Roleplay (Animal handling and customer communication).
- Ethics.
- Observational skills/large animal knowledge (this took place at the farm on the Harper-Adams campus).
- Practical aptitude test.
- Interpreting a mock consultation/chat about your personality and ability to handle stress.

Liverpool Institute of Veterinary Science

Overview
The University of Liverpool's first Veterinary School was the first of the UK Veterinary Schools to be part of a university, and the first to offer a degree in veterinary science. Building on this outstanding tradition, now the Institute of Veterinary Sciences, the Institute today has a continuing commitment to innovative veterinary education and research, giving students a fantastic start to their veterinary careers. Like many veterinary schools, Liverpool operates on a dual campus basis. One campus is located in the heart of Liverpool and this is where you will do the majority of your science and theory based learning for the first 3 years. The other campus (Leahurst), is the location of your year 4 and 5 studies and also the home of its world renowned equine centre.

Key points
- Leading equine centre
- Research-led teaching
- Prestigious university

How hard is it to get into Liverpool Vet School?
The Liverpool Institute of Veterinary Science (Livestock) is a highly competitive veterinary school, and the admission process is rigorous. The exact difficulty of getting into the school depends on a number of factors, including academic performance, extracurricular activities, and experience in the veterinary field.

For the Bachelor of Veterinary Science (BVSc) programme, applicants are expected to have achieved high grades at A-level or equivalent, with a strong emphasis on science subjects. The application process also involves submitting a personal statement and references, as well as attending an interview.

The selection process for the BVSc programme is highly competitive, and the school receives many more applications than it has places available. However, meeting the minimum academic requirements does not guarantee admission, as the school also considers factors such as personal qualities, work experience, and extracurricular activities.

Overall, getting into the Liverpool Institute of Veterinary Science is considered challenging, but not impossible. Students who have a strong academic record, relevant experience, and a passion for the field of veterinary science will have the best chance of success.

Teaching Style

Whilst it follows the traditional 3 years non-clinical 2 years clinical route, the university of Liverpool will teach your practical skills from day one by taking advantage of their facilities to develop handling and basic clinical skills such as suturing.

Teaching proper communication is of great importance to the institute therefore you will be putting this into practice with professional actors who act as your clients in simulated veterinary consultations. This is all built upon further in the second year and third year however the structure of teaching of year 3 integrates a research project, thus developing your research skills.

The variety of facilities at the veterinary campus (Leahurst) allows you to develop a healthy balance of skills in different veterinary areas. This is where you will learn during your fourth and fifth years and after the final exams you have the chance to choose an elective subject to study in greater depth allowing you to practise as a vet whilst benefiting from the support/expertise of the staff at the site.

University Life

The main campus, where you will spend your pre-clinical years, is located in the heart of the city of Liverpool - an incredibly vibrant, friendly and historical city. The Leahurst campus, located in the countryside surrounding Liverpool will be the location of your clinical years and consists of all things veterinary from its teaching animal hospitals to its leading equine centre. Not too far from each campus is Chester zoo which has strong ties with the university.

Liverpool is very well known for its entertaining night-life and since you'll be based in the heart of the city, you'll be in the centre of the fun. There's also a number of interesting scenic spots and historical locations which may interest you for a day out such as the Royal Albert Dock where you can find places like the Liverpool Tate art gallery and the Slavery Museum. You can also expect interesting excursions organised by the University itself which will take you all over the country.

Interview Style

Applicants will be invited to interview, which will take place sometime during November and December. The interviews will take the form of MMI stations. Interview topics include:
- Small Animal
- Large Animal
- Equine

Nottingham School of Veterinary Medicine and Science

Overview

Having set the example in the UK veterinary medicine scene of practical, hands-on, learning, the university of Nottingham will offer you the most extreme of this approach. Based on its own 'Sutton Bonington' Campus in the outskirts of Nottingham with its own, nearby working dairy farm and a plethora of clinical facilities such as a working teaching hospital on site, Nottingham veterinary school take practical learning a step further by introducing you to clinical examples and settings from day one so if you are keen hands-on learner then Nottingham is the place to be. In addition, this campus is the location of the majority of Nottingham's animal and agricultural science courses making it a fantastic centre for research thus allowing you to immerse yourself in various scientific projects.

Key points
- Day one clinical
- Relaxed on grades
- Two intakes

Insider's Guide to Nottingham Veterinary School

What makes Nottingham unique to other veterinary schools?

Nottingham definitely has the most practical course out of all of the other universities. You start gaining clinical exposure from your very first weeks. I find this aspect extremely helpful. It is a brilliant way to engage with the information that you are learning in lectures, and gradually start to apply it to clinical situations. For example, when learning about the anatomy of the forelimb, we would consolidate our knowledge by following content up with dissections. Being able to see the muscles and bones and understand where they are in 3D space is so helpful for learning anatomy. By the time that I have finished my first year, I will know how to do so many things that other vet schools only start teaching students during their clinical third years. It is a massive advantage. You start learning dissection techniques, clinical procedures, and animal handling skills immediately. For instance, I'm only in my eighth week of teaching, but we are already being exposed to MRI scans – something that a lot of vets may struggle with in practice!

So by the time that you finally reach your clinical years, you have a head-start above everybody else. You get so much practice at doing things like reading MRI scans, that you gradually start getting the hang of it.

And by the time that you graduate, you are more proficient at it than somebody who has had only two years to practise it.

Course Structure at Nottingham Veterinary School

Year 1: The main modules taught this year are the neuromuscular system and circulatory and respiratory systems, alongside animal health and welfare.

Year 2: The second year has a similar structure to Year 1, which the modules taught being the endocrine and integumentary system, urogenital system, and gastrointestinal system.

Year 3: The year begins with a short research project, followed by the beginning of clinical teaching.

Year 4: A year of clinical teaching, which immediately leads onto the 5th year when clinical rotations begin.

Year 5: An entire year of clinical rotations and elective weeks at the very end. There are no lectures during this academic year!

Teaching Style at Nottingham Veterinary School

Nottingham utilises a variety of teaching methods to ensure a holistic delivery of content. The main chunk of the content is delivered through a mixture of online and in-person lectures, all of which are recorded and always accessible to students. Other content is introduced through self-directed learning (SDL). This usually involves you being given a PowerPoint with guidance on what you need to learn. I have found the SDLs to be an absolutely brilliant way to develop my time management and research skills. As a graduate, you will regularly come across cases for which you may need to find more information. By developing these research skills early on, Nottingham vet students become very proficient at independently finishing their own resources out in practice. Furthermore, you get used to not having the answers given to you immediately, getting you used to uncertainty. This develops confidence in your own knowledge, ensuring that you can make decisions and trust yourself in the future.

Now onto one of my favourite parts of the course – the practicals. We have a minimum of one practical each week – it's usually two or three! This is used to consolidate knowledge of anatomy, imaging techniques, as well as learn clinical skills.

Small group teaching is used to consolidate and deepen our knowledge of what we learn throughout the week, as well as improve awareness of ethics and topical issues.

This is a brilliant way to meet people and develop your ability to communicate effectively with each other. Finally, regular workshops and wrap-up sessions are opportunities to consolidate the content on an almost weekly basis. These tend to be interactive and Q&A sessions with a fun Kahoot to mix things up!

University Life

Despite Sutton Bonington (SB) being a 30 minutes bus ride away from the main campus in Nottingham's city centre, there is still plenty to do on campus! There are a variety of societies and sports clubs dedicated solely to students studying on SB. My favourite activity is climbing. It's a brilliant way to both enjoy yourself and meet so many new people! Unfortunately, there aren't quite as many sports clubs at SB as there are on the main campus. This can prove to be a bit tricky for people who want to participate in competitive sports that only run on the main campus. Some people decide to live in the accommodation there instead, despite it meaning that they have to travel to lectures every day. Otherwise, getting from SB to the main campus is very easy – you can even do some work on the bus!

As I'm not somebody who enjoys clubbing or partying, I wouldn't be able to comment on what that aspect of the social life on SB looks like! What's great, is that if you're someone like me, there are still social events to get involved in that don't involve drinking or loud music. The campus regularly hosts dining evenings, pub quizzes, movie nights, games evenings, and much more. There's something to get involved in for everyone! The vet school also runs several veterinary societies. The one I'm most active in is the Surgical Society. And it's awesome! I've only been to a few sessions so far, but I have learnt how to correctly use equipment, suturing techniques, and even got to practise my new skills on some pork bellies! It's a brilliant society to get involved in if you're interested in surgery like I am.

Interview Style

Additional assessment may include interviews or tests. Some courses may ask for examples of written work. Where courses use additional assessment, admissions staff send information to applicants, explaining the nature of the assessment, what admissions staff will be looking for and how applicants can prepare. If applicants are invited to interview, this will be a panel interview. Common interview topics include:

- Group challenges.
- Practical assessment.
- Personal Statement.
- Ethics.
- Motivation and insight into the course.
- How you deal with stress.
- Knowledge of the veterinary world.
- Communication skills.

Royal Veterinary College London

Overview
At arguably the most prestigious veterinary school in the UK, the Bachelor of Veterinary Medicine programme offered by RVC offers world-leading scientific and clinical training in veterinary medicine. RVC is located in the heart of London (Camden) and offers a vast range of veterinary programmes (from veterinary nursing to postgraduate veterinary degrees. Their Veterinary Medicine and Surgery degree, however, is a course built upon their extensive veterinary history, and takes a fresh approach in bringing together technological change, clinical and scientific progress, and stimulating teaching and learning methods.

Key points
- London
- Global accreditation
- Prestigious

Insider's Guide to RVC School

What makes RVC unique to other veterinary schools?
What really stood out to me about the RVC when I was applying for vet med was how passionate RVC students are about the university. Now as an RVC student myself I completely understand this love for the university. It is an incredible university to be a student at because all of the students are so friendly. Some people think that being at a university of just vet students would be boring but this couldn't be further from the truth. We are all linked by our shared goal of being vets and this creates an incredible community to be a part of. Something else that makes the RVC really stand out is that it is accredited in the UK, the EU and the USA and Canada. This gives students the option to work in these countries much more easily when they qualify which will open endless opportunities to travel and gain experience abroad.

How hard is it to get into Royal Veterinary College?
Admission to the Royal Veterinary College (RVC) is highly competitive, and the selection process is rigorous. The RVC is one of the leading veterinary schools in the United Kingdom, and its programs are highly sought after.

The admission process takes into account a range of factors, including academic achievement, work experience, and personal statement.

To be considered for admission to the RVC, applicants are required to meet a number of requirements, including a strong academic background in science or a related field.

In addition, applicants must have relevant work experience, a compelling personal statement, and pass an interview process.

The number of spaces available in each program is limited, and the admission process is highly competitive. As such, getting into the Royal Veterinary College can be challenging, and applicants are encouraged to carefully review the requirements and prepare thoroughly for the application process. However, with hard work, dedication, and a strong application, it is possible to gain admission to the RVC and pursue a rewarding career in veterinary medicine or biosciences.

Course Structure at RVC School

The RVC uses a spiral curriculum which means that topics you cover in first year will come up in subsequent years where they will be developed on and become increasingly more complex in different contexts. The first 2 years are preclinical so here you learn about the healthy animal so that in years 3-5 you can learn about what is abnormal.

Year 1 at RVC School
In the first year you learn about the main body systems such as the locomotor strand (which is learning about how the animal moves, the limbs etc.) and the alimentary strand (which is all about the digestive system). This is where you learn about the basic principles that can then be developed with clinical knowledge later in the course. There are weekly practicals to help with learning anatomy.

Year 2 at RVC School
Second year is the last pre-clinical year so in this year you will revisit many of the strands from last year to add detail and complexity to these principles. There are more practicals and dissections too to help learn the anatomy of the normal, healthy animal.

Year 3 at RVC School
Third year is the first clinical year so this is where you will begin to learn about diseases and how these can be treated.

Year 4 at RVC School
Fourth year contains some teaching and also clinical rotations which is where you will spend time out in clinics observing consultations and surgeries to put all of your learning into practice and expand upon it.

Year 5 at RVC School
Fifth year you also spend doing your clinical rotations.

Teaching Style

The RVC has lots of group work so we complete a directed learning every week which is where you work through a task with your tutor group. This may be a clinical case or something similar where you use the lectures from the week to put that knowledge into practice and use the information to problem solve. These sessions are really helpful in making content make sense and helping you to remember what you have been taught. We also have weekly practicals to help us learn anatomy which is really helpful as things look very different in the real animal to in pictures online!

The RVC does have a lot of dissection which is really helpful for starting to learn how to properly hold and use surgical instruments before we even get to the clinical years. It is also really helpful in learning the anatomy of the animals.

University Life

RVC teaching centre and living halls are located in Camden in the heart of London and the home to well-known locations such as Camden Market and London Zoo. Like many of the other Veterinary Schools, you will find everything you need on campus and your flats will only be a short distance away from here. The Hawkshead campus (based in Hertfordshire) will feature a more peaceful, countryside area - perfect for the practical/clinical training you will be undergoing in these final 3 years.

A visit to the nearby bustling Camden Market or ZSL London Zoo is a great way to spend your day locally. However, you'll be in the centre of London thus leaving you either walking distance or a short underground journey away from an excess of attractions, restaurants, pubs, bars and nightclubs so night/day life will not be a problem.

Furthermore, despite its relatively small scale in comparison to other universities, you will not fall short in terms of sports clubs and societies and if you can't find one for you, feel free to start up your own.

Interview Style

The RVC conducts their interviews in the form of MMI stations and an observed group task. Interviews commonly take place between November and December.

Surrey School of Veterinary Medicine

Overview
The University of Surrey will offer you a course with an emphasis on a practical hands-on approach to learning. This is accomplished through the utilisation of its state of the art animal handling teaching facility and its second to none partner networking scheme which connects you with a plethora of industry links, real working animal environments and incredible placement opportunities which you will be free to make the most of. In addition, with its leading research facilities, Surrey pays particular attention to laboratory work, thus will teach you a superior level of laboratory based skills which will undoubtedly make you stand out from the crowd in the veterinary world, upon graduation.

Key points
- Vast partner-network scheme
- Modern facilities
- High student satisfaction

Teaching Style
Surrey's Veterinary Medicine course follows the traditional route meaning the first 3 years are non-clinical, consisting mostly of animal handling training, lab training and theory. Only in years 4 and 5 will you begin your clinical work. However, throughout the first 3 years you will be taught mostly in a practical manner that will take full advantage of their research facilities and their vast partner networking scheme giving you the opportunity to learn practically in realistic working animal environments.

University Life
The veterinary medicine course is located on one of the two campuses which are approximately 5 minutes walking distance from each other. Everything you need for your course can be found on-campus however you may be living in either of these 2 picturesque locations. The surrounding area is the city of guildford based in the heart of Surrey.

The University of Surrey boasts a new, state of the art sports centre with facilities for a huge variety of different activities so if you are that-way inclined you can be sure Surrey will satisfy.

In the surrounding area, Guildford, you will find plenty of vibrant pubs, bars and clubs to entertain you on your nights out along with a fantastic live-music venue, G-Live, which attracts many world renowned artists year-round.

Interview Style

The University of Surrey invites successful applicants to take part in MMI stations. There are typically eight stations, with a time-limit of 6 minutes each. The interviews are held between November and January. Common MMI topics include:
- Ethical Station
- Roleplay (Teaching)
- Workplace situational problem solving
- Professionalism in the workplace
- Outside of the box (unpredictable)
- Roleplay (hypothetical situational problem solving)
- Personality Questionnaire

Teaching Styles

You may have noticed that there are differences in the teaching styles offered across vet schools. Before your interview make sure to research the vet school's syllabus and find out about the type of course they offer.

It is very common to be asked about the vet school's curriculum in your interview. It is expected that consideration of teaching style will have been a key factor in your decision to apply to that particular vet school. The interviewers are looking for you to be knowledgeable about their curriculum and to demonstrate that you are well suited to the style of teaching.

Common Pitfall
Remember to explain to the interviewer why your skills complement the curriculum. You need to convince the panel their teaching style is well fitting to you. Avoid simply listing elements of the curriculum without explaining why each aspect would benefit your learning overall.

Spiral/strand learning

Spiral or strand learning is common in a lot of vet schools given the preclinical to clinical year learning difference. It refers to learning the basics for one subject (for example locomotor) in year 1, then developing more on that and only revisiting it in year 2. You will then revisit it in years 3-4 where you will learn what can go wrong with locomotion and how this can be resolved clinically.

An advantage of strand based learning is that you are not overwhelmed with too much information at one given time. Strand based learning allows vet students to constantly be referring and integrating their theory knowledge into clinical settings in later years up until actual vet work post graduation.

Anatomy Teaching

Anatomy is taught during the preclinical phase of a veterinary degree. The topic of anatomy is taught in a variety of ways with a surprising amount of variation in teaching methods between UK vet schools. Anatomy is traditionally one of the toughest aspects of veterinary medicine for first-year students, so it is worth researching the teaching at your chosen universities.

Dissection

Cadaveric dissection is the traditional method of teaching anatomy to vet students. It involves cutting a body specimen to reveal anatomical structures to aid learning. Vet schools utilising dissection will expect students to carry out the dissection themselves, often in small groups, using animal cadavers.

Dissection is a very hands-on approach and allows students to see, physically touch, and explore organs to further their learning.

Prosection
In contrast to traditional dissection, prosection involves students examining pre-prepared cadaveric samples. This means all of the cutting and dissection is performed by trained anatomists instead of students themselves. The major advantage of this is the high quality of dissection which can make it easier to identify important structures.

Prosection is becoming increasingly favoured by vet schools, as it is a more time efficient method of teaching. Students also have the opportunity to examine samples from multiple cadavers and can more easily gain an appreciation of normal anatomical variations.

Rotations
During your 4th year and into 5th year you will be placed into small groups - this is your rotation group. During rotations, you and your group will work together as a team during clinical rounds in different settings such as hospitals or on farms.

Your rotation group is a good way to apply how you should be working in a team as you will eventually be doing this once a practising vet.

Other styles of learning
Vet schools are constantly updating their curriculum and new teaching styles are emerging each year. For example, in recent years some universities have introduced blended learning referring to lectures done in one's own time alongside in person scheduled lecturers.
Regardless of the teaching style, remember to thoroughly research the course structure and prepare a handful of key benefits ready to discuss at interview. You should do this for each individual vet school and be specific to each course.

Chapter 2: Work Experience

Work Experience Introduction

Work experience in the context of vet school admissions can be defined as any type of activity or life experience which has prepared you for a veterinary medicine career in some way. Although vet schools generally appreciate that work experience can be difficult to obtain, particularly since the pandemic, most vet schools require a minimum number of hours and for you to do certain types of work experience.

For example, RVC currently requires applicants to obtain a total of 70 hours (10 full days) of work experience in one or more veterinary practices, as well as 70 hours in one or more non-clinical working environments with live animals.

You will likely be asked about your work experience directly at an interview with questions such as "*What was your favourite part of your work experience?*" However, this is not the only time work experience can be incorporated in your answer. It may be useful to consider work experience as **evidence** that you can use to strengthen most answers. For example, a strong answer to the question "*What are the challenges of working as a vet?*" will use observations from their work experience to support any points made. Try and show off all the interesting work experience you have completed whenever it is relevant!

Why do we need work experience?

There are a number of reasons why vet schools ask applicants to carry out work experience placements, including:

- Gaining a **realistic** understanding of veterinary medicine, including the physical demands of the job, organisation of the clinical environment, and emotional demands of the career.
- Developing values and skills essential to becoming a vet, including communication, teamwork and empathy. We will explore this further in the 'Personal Qualities and Skills' section of this book.
- Demonstrating motivation and commitment to a career in veterinary medicine, which is particularly applicable to long-term placements requiring a significant time commitment.

Keeping these three points in mind when talking about work experience at your interviews will ensure you are providing examples relevant to the competencies interviewers are assessing.

Getting started

When you are conducting your work experience it is useful to keep a diary of your observations and review this prior to any interviews. Similarly, some students like to create a mind map of each placement to reflect on what they saw and learnt and how this could be applied to potential interview questions.

You should aim to have a set of well thought-out and reflected points developed from your work experience that you are prepared to mention in multiple interview scenarios.

Interview Tip
You will not have time to mention every interesting aspect of every work experience placement you have carried out. Be selective about what scenarios you discuss and make sure these are those that display the highest quality reflections. It is much easier to do this if you have prepared in advance.

Small Animal Work Experience

Work experience at a small animal clinic is where most vet applicants start as the basis of the application. Shadowing a small animal veterinary surgeon is a good way to get an idea of the life of a vet given that nearly 70% of graduates chose this path. More importantly, first opinion small animal practices are where most pets will end up when they first become unwell or have been scheduled for appointments.

What can I expect from small animal work experience?

No two work experience placements are the same and you are not expected to see a minimum number of consultations or complete a set list of activities. However, if you mention undertaking a small animal clinical work experience placement you could be asked about specific aspects of GP care as it is expected that you will have observed, or discussed, common activities that GPs perform during their daily work.

Take a look at your work experience diary and try to find examples where you observed the following aspects of small animal veterinary care.

Same day or emergency appointments

These are for patients who need to be seen urgently and are typically booked into a number of empty slots, kept aside and awaiting a triage approach to fitting them into the daily schedule. Sometimes other veterinarians may also book patients at the end of their clinics too - how do you think they manage this in terms of timing?

Pre-booked or routine appointments

These are for patients with non-urgent problems who can wait days to weeks for appointment slots.

This could be used for medication reviews, following-up chronic diseases and delivering routine test results. Did you observe any differences in the types of conditions seen at these appointments?

Telephone consultations
Telephone consultations are being utilised increasingly in both primary and secondary care settings. Can you think of any limitations or benefits of this? If you observed a telephone consultation, think about how the vet adapted their communication style compared to a traditional face-to-face appointment.

Additionally, think about which member of the veterinary clinic team took this call - can you say anything about the importance of this and how triaging works in a small animal clinic?

Nurse appointments
Following on from this, sitting in on nurse clinics is a great way to understand the differences between the job roles of vet nurses and vets. Think about any differences you observed - was this what you expected? You may find nurses carry out more traditional 'vet jobs' than you initially expected! How did this influence your motivation to study veterinary medicine?

Reception work
You may have been presented with the opportunity to sit with a vet receptionist. This provides an appreciation of the impact non-clinical staff can have on patient and client care. Can you think of any examples of good care or communication provided by one of the receptionists?

Surgical Work Experience

During your small-animal first opinion clinic experience it is more than likely you got to see some surgeries. Most of this will be regular routine surgeries such as neutering or dental work however do include handling some traumatic injuries. Surgery is a key part to being a vet of any kind since as a vet you will be expected to be always involved in surgery no matter the animal or issue at hand.

What can I expect from surgical work experience?

Observing operations
Witnessing operations is probably the aspect of surgery that students look forward to the most. Operations can either be performed as an emergency or elective, meaning they have been planned in advance.

Common pitfall
Remember that work experience is not about what you have done, but rather what you learnt and took away from the experience. Interviewers will not be fooled by candidates who simply list complex procedures they have witnessed in a bid to be impressive. Instead, reflect on the experience including simple interactions between colleagues.

Members of the surgical team

Thinking of a routine spay, the surgical team will consist of the main veterinary surgeon and usually one veterinary nurse. Try and talk to both of these staff members if possible to understand what their role is during surgery and how it impacts the patient and how their owner might be feeling.

Chapter 3: Applying to Veterinary Medicine

UCAS Veterinary Application Guide 2024

Considering a career as a vet? You will need to apply to study Veterinary Medicine and you can do this via UCAS, the Universities and Colleges Admissions Service. Read on for all the information you need to apply for 2025 entry.

What is the UCAS Application for Veterinary Medicine?
If you are applying to study veterinary medicine at a college or university in the UK, you need to do this through UCAS. They manage all UK applications for higher education. The good thing about applying through UCAS is that they will send your application to all the institutions you have applied to so you don't need to do it!

What Is Included in the UCAS Veterinary Application?
There are a number of things you must consider to help make your UCAS Veterinary application stand out:
- Work Experience
- Application Questions
- Veterinary Personal Statement
- Supplementary Assessment Questionnaire (SAQs) – Selected schools
- Veterinary Interview

In addition to the above, if you are planning on studying veterinary medicine at the University of Cambridge, you will be required to sit the Engineering and Science Admissions Test (ESAT). Please note, that the ESAT replaces the Natural Sciences Aptitude Assessment (NSAA) from 2024.

Important UCAS Dates for 2025 Entry
Veterinary applications are required to be submitted earlier than an application to study other courses.

<u>The UCAS Veterinary Deadline for 2024 entry is 16 October 2024 at 18:00. For up-to-date information on dates, please refer to the UCAS website.</u>

What does it Cost to Study Veterinary Medicine in the UK?
If you are a resident in England or Wales, veterinary courses can cost up to £9,250 per year. If you are a Scottish resident, you can study in Scotland for free. Costs for students studying in Northern Ireland will vary and are also dependent on where you live.

However, if you are an international student wishing to study in the UK, costs can be much higher; between £20000 to £45000 a year.

Financial Aid to Study Veterinary Medicine

If you are a UK or EU resident, you can apply for a loan to cover the costs of your course. This can be applied for via the government's student finance website. You can also check to see if you are eligible to apply for a loan to support you in financing your cost of living. In addition to this, check with the universities you are applying to as some of them also offer their own financial aid for students.

UCAS Application Cost

A registration fee is applicable when applying to study veterinary medicine through UCAS. The cost for this is £20 if you are applying to a single university course or £25 for multiple courses. Check with your school as they may pay this fee for you.

How many veterinary courses can I apply to?

When applying for courses through UCAS, you can apply to a maximum of 5 courses. However, only 4 of these can be veterinary medicine.

You can apply for a fifth non-veterinary course. With veterinary medicine being very competitive, it is highly recommended to have a fallback plan just in case.

How hard is it to get into veterinary school?

As we alluded to before, places on veterinary courses are very sought after and therefore, veterinary medicine is very competitive.

It is vital that you stand out from the crowd and the first step is through your UCAS veterinary application. This is your first chance to make a good impression. Read our step-by-step guide below for more information.

The UCAS Veterinary Application: A Step-by-Step Approach

1. School Exams

When you have decided to pursue a career in the veterinary profession, it is important to choose the right exams to study. Many universities have entry requirements when it comes to exams needed and many will also specify exams that are also favourable.

The next step is to score highly in those exams, particularly Biology and Chemistry.

2. Veterinary School Selection

As the decision of which exams to take will be based on requirements of different schools, you will have no doubt already started to think about this even before step 1.

When selecting veterinary schools for application, it is important to look at the type of course and teaching methods and think about whether it is a good fit for you. Location may also be an important factor. Attending Open Days and requesting prospectuses will help you narrow down your selection.

3. Work Experience

Work experience is an important part of the veterinary school application. Not only does it help to confirm that you want to study towards a career as a vet, but it will also show institutions that you are serious about your choice and have considered and experienced different aspects of the veterinary profession.

It is also important to note that if you are successful in securing an interview at one or more vet schools, part of your interview will focus on the work experience you have undertaken.

4. Medical Admissions Tests – ONLY For Cambridge Applications

Students are not required to take a standardised medical admissions test when applying to study veterinary medicine.

The one exception to this is students that apply to the University of Cambridge to study veterinary medicine. Students will be required to sit the Engineering and Science Admissions Test (ESAT). This takes place on 15 and 16 October 2024.

5. UCAS Personal Statement

As part of your UCAS medicine application, you will need to provide a veterinary personal statement to support your application.

The schools that you apply to will use this as part of the interview selection process. The personal statement limit is only 4000 characters long and so it is important to structure your personal statement in a way that makes you stand out from the crowd.

6. UCAS Application Submission

When you have gathered all the required information, you will submit your veterinary applications to UCAS. Remember that the deadline for veterinary applications is before the deadline for other courses. Your application will not be accepted after this deadline.

6a. Supplementary Assessment Questionnaire – Selected Schools

After you have submitted your UCAS application, selected schools may send you an SAQ to complete. The questions are based on your personality, work experience and personal qualities.

7. Veterinary School Interviews

Once you have submitted your UCAS veterinary application, you will need to wait to hear from veterinary schools regarding interviews. It is important to check the vet school website as to the timeline for contacting students regarding an interview and how they will be communicating this to them. Some schools send emails, some vis post and some through the UCAS portal. You can expect to hear about interviews from November, with interviews taking place between December and March.

After this, you will need to prepare for your veterinary interview. Research whether the interview will be a panel interview or an MMI (mini medical interviews), where there will be several stations to visit and answer questions on. Preparing for your veterinary interview is important. This is your last chance to make a good impression and stand out from the competition.

8. Veterinary School Offers

After the interviews comes more waiting! Schools will usually contact students within a month with a decision and the timeline will be published on their website.

Celebrations will ensue and you will be on your way to becoming a veterinary professional!

Chapter 4: Veterinary Personal Statement

Veterinary Personal Statement: The Introduction

The first few lines of your personal statement is the first impression that admissions tutors will have of you. It is very daunting to begin writing your personal statement, especially when you place so much emphasis on it. Here are some top tips for writing your veterinary personal statement introduction.

Write the introduction last
It might seem logical to start writing your Veterinary Personal Statement from the beginning, brainstorming introduction starters. However, the introduction is arguably the most difficult paragraph to write. Many students fixate on writing a "killer opening line", if you overthink your introduction, you may end up procrastinating from tackling the rest of your Veterinary Personal Statement. If you find that you are struggling with crafting an introduction, then it might be better to start writing the other sections (such as work experience or talking about your personal achievements) first.

Make it Personal
When describing your motivation for studying Veterinary think about what you have learnt about *being* a vet and then *why* you want to be a vet. The introduction should be based around your personal motivation to study Veterinary Medicine, so avoid making your reasons generic.

Grip the reader immediately
The introduction of your Veterinary Personal Statement should be the first thing to grasp the reader's attention, make it snappy and captivating. This is the difference between your application grabbing someone's attention and it being like all the others they have read. Use your judgement to assess whether your opening lines are authentic and personal to you.

Show an understanding of Veterinary as a degree and profession
It is important to demonstrate that you understand what a career in Veterinary Medicine involves. Do not fall into the trap of describing your "love for cuddling animals." This phrase will make the reader question if you are aware of what the job actually involves (it actually involves quite little of this). There are difficult, messy, and upsetting parts to the job.

The Veterinary Schools Council Website provides excellent information about careers and admissions into Vet School.

Common Pitfalls in a Veterinary Personal Statement Introduction

Using Clichés
Avoid sounding cliché and using phrases such as 'I love animals and science.' This is a hackneyed phrase that will not make you stand out. The word "Passion" croups up lots of times in Veterinary Personal Statements. Passion is an emotion… and it does not fit well describing your chosen career as an emotive feeling. Lastly, avoid using the word 'dream' and saying, 'veterinary medicine is my dream'. This may be the case, but if you mention this it doesn't come across as very professional, and can sound like you're unaware of the realities of the profession.

Using unnatural language
Using flowery and verbose language will not impress the admissions tutor. By using unnatural language, it immediately looks like you have used a thesaurus to change up your words. A common example of this is using the word 'relish' to describe how much you like doing something. You may want to use synonyms to avoid repeating words. Make sure if that you are still using appropriate concise words in their correct context.

Using Sob Stories
You can use personal anecdotes to help explain your reasoning for wanting to study Veterinary Medicine. Be careful not to make these sound too cliché. Steer away from phrases such as 'When I was 5 I had a pet hamster that became sick and its treatment at the vets is what inspired me to become one'.

Being Generic
Mentioning that you like science can be another common pitfall in Veterinary Personal Statement introductions. Veterinary medicine combines science and a love of working with animals' hand in hand. Try to be original when explaining why you like the science aspect of the job. What specifically do you enjoy? How have you had experience of veterinary science in your schooling? e.g. dissections in class or learning about the heart can relate a lot to veterinary anatomy.

N.B. – Do not let the fear of sounding too generic put you off from mentioning animals at all in your introduction. If you are studying to be a vet, you should like animals and you should talk about them in your Veterinary Personal Statement. Try to individually explain why you like them, what is it about working with them that you enjoy? Why is studying veterinary medicine a good choice for you given that you like animals?

A Veterinary Personal Statement Introduction Idea

Consider beginning your Veterinary Personal Statement describing a particular 'ology' that you have enjoyed learning about or researching. Think about how you can use this to explain why you want to be a vet. For example, you may describe that you have an interest in cardiology, because you've seen a cardio case on your Veterinary work experience. Did this inspire you to look into the future of veterinary cardiology?

Veterinary Personal Statement: Academic Interests

It is a great idea to talk about your academic interests in your Veterinary Personal Statement. Use your Personal Statement as an opportunity to show off your aptitude for science. Veterinary degrees are academically demanding, and the career involves lifelong learning. Therefore, admissions tutors are looking to identify students who can show that they are curious and dedicated to academia.

Common Questions: Academic Interests

Why is it important to discuss your academic interests?
Reflecting and describing your academic interests in your Veterinary Personal Statement allows you to show what extra efforts you're making to widen your knowledge outside of the taught curriculum. This will help you stand out from other applicants.

What do we mean by "Academic Interests?"
When we talk about academic interests, what this refers to is anything that you may have achieved in school that does not include your A level or GCSE grades. Please do not waste characters putting your grades into your Veterinary Personal Statement.

Examples of super-curricular activities/ academic achievements:
The sorts of academic achievements that you could write about include the following:
- Sponsored reads/book clubs that you are part of
- Debating societies
- Interests in science or veterinary medicine from reading magazines such as 'In Practice' 'The Vet Times' or online journals
- Journal clubs at your school
- Extended Project qualifications
- Books that you've read

Common pitfalls when describing your academic achievements

Lying
Do not lie within this section of your Veterinary Personal Statement (or in any other section). If you state that you have read something or won an award... please ensure this is true. At Veterinary MMI/ Panel interviews they may ask about your academic interests and what you have written about them. It would be embarrassing if you did not know what they were talking about or didn't know how to answer their questions.

Listing
Never just list facts about yourself in your Veterinary Personal Statement.

Stating not explaining
Do not just state your academic achievements but put them into context. Consider what you learnt and how this will help you in your career as a vet.

We have shown you a good and bad example of this is practice:

> Bad Example – 'I was part of my schools Oxbridge society'

> Good Example: 'Being selected to be part of my school's Oxbridge society has allowed me to have access to a plethora of scientific journals in which I have been able to research my interest in veterinary microbiology more thoroughly'. I found X interesting and am looking forward to expanding my knowledge on this throughout vet school.'

In the second example can you see that the student presents the achievement in a constructive way rather than just stating their achievements.

Sweeping Statements
Academic awards are great tangible achievements to write about in your Veterinary Personal Statement. You may have gained awards for the most improved grade or an award for your continued efforts towards your studies – these are great things to put in! A pitfall is describing ranking highly in your year group using a sweeping statement – many students may describe coming "near the top" of their year group.

Your Veterinary Personal Statement should contain solid evidence, not sweeping statements about achievements relative to those of others.

Top tips for Writing About Your Academic Interests

1. Planning is essential!

Ensure you know which academic interests you want to write about and consider which paragraph these reflections fit in with. We advise that it is best to write about any personal or academic achievements in your penultimate/ last paragraph. It is always good to end with reflections on what else you do outside of your normal teaching and hobbies.

2. Show Proactivity and an interest in Veterinary

It is a good idea to talk about your achievements, or something interesting you have read and link it back to how this can benefit you during your time at vet school.

For example, imagine that you are writing about your extended project on badger culling due to TB. How could you relate this to a career in veterinary medicine? You could describe your understanding of the large debate as to whether badgers do spread the disease or not. It would be good to include any interesting points from your research that you found out here and expand on them for future development. For example you may have come across research into a vaccine for TB in the future from your EPQ research. You could mention that this would be an interesting area to learn about at vet school in the coming years as the evidence is continually changing.

So, whatever your academic achievements may be (and believe me everyone will have at least one they should be able to think of), always remember to include them in your Veterinary Personal Statement.

Veterinary Personal Statement: Extra-Curricular Activities

The concept of having a good work-life balance is becoming increasingly important as part of the Veterinary student selection process. In your Veterinary Personal Statement, it is vital to reference your extra-curricular activities as these can help you to display that you have developed the skills and attributes needed by vets. Hobbies show that you have a good work-life balance and that you would continue to have a life out of vet school so please don't forget to include them as they are very important things that universities look for.

Structuring your Veterinary Personal Statement

You might be wondering where it is best to write about extracurricular activities in your personal statement. Ultimately, the decision is up to you where you choose to include it.

We recommend students use the following structure and therefore reference their extracurricular activities in the last few paragraphs:
- An introduction explaining their motivations to study Veterinary medicine.
- A middle paragraph explaining about work experience.
- A paragraph (or two) at the end where you talk about your personal achievements, hobbies, academic achievements etc.

How much of your Veterinary Personal Statement should be dedicated to your extracurricular activities?

Our top tip when writing about your extracurricular activities is to keep it brief. Your personal statement should be academically focused. Most of your characters should describe why you want to study veterinary and why the university should offer you a place at Veterinary school. Work experience and your knowledge and interest in the subject should contribute more to the content of your veterinary personal statement that your extracurriculars paragraph.

What to include in your paragraph about extracurricular activities

Extra-curricular is quite an umbrella term which might have you wondering what you should include as part of this. Broadly speaking, extra-curricular activities include any part time jobs you may have/ volunteering that you do, any particular programmes that you may have participated in (eg PGL or NCS), and any hobbies that you may have.

In a nutshell, this is everything that you do that is non-academic and not work experience that you feel has made an impact in making you a good candidate to apply to vet school.

If you have lots of hobbies and extra-curricular activities, then you may struggle to write about all of these in your application. If this is the case, cherry-pick the most important ones to you or the ones that you can easily relate to making you more skilled to being a vet.

Below is a comprehensive list of extra-curricular activities that you may want to include in your application:
- Duke of Edinburgh award
- School clubs e.g., debating clubs/ societies.
- Private tutoring
- Part time jobs e.g., paper rounds/ retail work/ hospitality etc
- Volunteering positions e.g., caring for the elderly or volunteering at an animal charity
- PGL trips
- School prefect
- National Citizen Service (NCS) summer programmes
- Camp America etc
- School trips away e.g., to Kenya wildlife reserves
- Charity events for animal foundations e.g., sponsored runs
- Hobbies
- Musical instruments and their grading
- Sports

How to write about your extracurricular activities in your Veterinary Personal Statement

When writing about your extracurricular activities, it is important not to just list them, but to always relate them back to how they will impact you as a vet/ vet student.

Think about what you have learnt from these activities, or how they have developed you as a person, whether this is through teamwork, improving communication skills, improving your ability to rationalise and prioritise decisions etc. All of these skills are so broad and can be developed from nearly all tasks if you think about it, so do try to say what you've learnt from each activity individually. However, in the part where you write about your hobbies, it's okay if you do not relate these directly to veterinary, but instead you could mention that you have maintained a good work-life balance through doing these hobbies instead and are aware of how important this is to being a vet alongside clinical work.

Check out the UCAS official guidance on writing about your hobbies in your Personal Statement.

Good and Bad examples of extracurricular activity reflections

Below are some examples of how you can talk about extra-curricular activities and what makes these good/ bad:

'In my free time I like to play netball which has improved my teamwork skills.'

Picking apart this sentence an admission tutor would certainly question the student's phrasing. Within the first 15 characters the student has already raised alarm bells to the reader by describing how they have 'free time.' If possible, avoid this phrase! But why? Time is of the essence in vet school, and even as a student you're busy a lot of the time. Vet school is difficult to get into and requires a lot of prep… meaning your time is valuable and not free by any means!

Think about how you would reword this sentence. How about using phrases such as 'In my spare time,' or 'in my downtime from my studies' etc.

What else could this student do to improve? The student needs to add some meat to the bones of their answer to show enthusiasm and passion. This student has explained the hobby and how it has helped them develop a skill (improved teamwork skills), but they could have expanded on this. Consider why this hobby may potentially help our student when practising and studying veterinary.

> 'In my downtime from my studies I play netball for my school team. This has helped me to improve my teamwork skills by enhancing my communication and ability to work well with different individuals, which I can draw many parallels to when working in a veterinary team with nurses and vets.'

We're starting to see some improvement in this student's work. They've mentioned they still have a life outside of schoolwork, but they're still not showing how their extracurricular activities have helped them develop attributes needed by those working in a veterinary environment.

> 'My participation in the National citizen service scheme has shown my determination by using my summer holidays to fully immerse myself into unknown challenges, and remain calm, which will benefit me as a vet student when it comes to dealing with cases where I am unsure of what is wrong with the animal.'

By draft three they have cracked it and produced a good paragraph. They've listed the extra-curricular, listed the skill they've improved and then shown how that can relate to veterinary.So, what can we learn from this student?

We want you to be using the formula used by the student in the third example. This is the kind of formula you should use when talking about all your extra-curricular activities.

Veterinary Personal Statement: The Conclusion

Effectively concluding your Veterinary Personal Statement is very important as a way to nicely round off what you have written. How you end your Veterinary Personal statement is going to leave a lasting impression in the reader's mind about how your whole statement.

When coming to write the conclusion, you may realise you are close to the character or maximum line limit, ending abruptly without a thorough conclusion is a common personal statement pitfall.

In addition to our tips below, the UCAS website has also compiled some generic but useful advice for ending your Personal Statement.

Tips for ending and concluding your personal statement

1. Keep it brief and do not waffle

Your conclusion should not be too long, only a few lines.

2. Show Veterinary is right for you and focus on personal motivation

Your conclusion should reiterate why you want to study Veterinary Medicine. You should summarise how your skill set will make you a good vet. Try to sell yourself and show the admissions tutor why they should offer you a place.

3. Avoid Repetition

Try not to directly repeat phrases that you have already mentioned previously in your Veterinary Personal Statement. This wastes valuable characters.

4. Tie is back to what you have written earlier

It is ok to reference and repeat the skills described within the body of the personal statement. However, use a different choice of words so that it does not look like you have just lifted the same information from your introduction or main body paragraphs.

5. Ensure your conclusion has a focus on the Veterinary world and science

You could use your conclusion to reference the future of Veterinary medicine. Consider the following question: what is it about today's society or the future of veterinary medicine that inspires you to want to be part of this career?

Walkthrough Examples: Concluding your Veterinary Personal Statement

We have written an example of an excellent concluding paragraph:

'Nowadays the combination of human science and medicine with that of veterinary medicine has opened a whole new range of treatment methods that can benefit our pets. In particular, with the introduction of prosthetic implants for orthopaedic injuries, I am intrigued to learn what the future of veterinary medicine will hold at the rate it is progressing, and want to be a part of creating these new innovations to better the lives of animals and humans.'

This is a very good answer because the student's motivation for wanting to study Veterinary Medicine shines through. For example, they have shown awareness that by bettering the lives of animals, they are bettering the lives of humans too. Moreover, the student shows that they understand the parallels between veterinary and human medicine. They acknowledge that (although veterinary medicine is about 30 years behind human medicine), we can achieve great things from a combined approach.

The student rounds off the statement nicely avoiding being too abrupt. This brings the statement to a close with an all-encompassing feeling that they have fully explained why they would be a good vet student.

Veterinary Personal Statement: Wider Reading

In preparation for your Veterinary application, you may have been told that you need to do some "wider reading." It can be difficult to know what to read, how much to read and how to approach writing about what you have read in your Veterinary Personal Statement. Within this article we aim to outline why reading books and engaging in projects, or societies will boost your Veterinary application.

Common Questions: Wider Reading

What do we mean by "Wider Reading"?
Wider reading involves going off to research or read about a topic that is not part of your national. It involves personal efforts to go and learn more about a topic that you may have particular interest in.

Why do I need to do wider reading?
Wider reading allows students to actively demonstrate an interest in Veterinary. Reading is an excellent way to explore your interest in science and the career. By reading you can build up an accurate representation of what being a Veterinary professional is really like. The point of showing that you have done wider reading is to show you have put the effort in to research a topic you've probably stumbled across and found interesting and wanted to learn more about.

What are some examples of wider veterinary reading?
Examples of wider reading that you may include in your personal statement involve:
- Scientific journals (such as those found on pub med, google scholar etc)
- Magazine articles (be careful and only use official veterinary magazines eg In practice or Vet Record).
- Books (any veterinary anatomy books such as Dyce, Konig etc) or you may have other veterinary physiology books you can reference.
- Internet articles (be VERY careful about saying that you have read something on the internet without being sure it's from an accredited source. You do not want to be referencing a Facebook comment!)

Check out the introductory reading list created by the University of Cambridge Department of Veterinary Medicine for ideas of where to start with your reading.

Help! I have not read any Veterinary books…
Wider reading is not essential for having a successful veterinary application. If you have not researched anything or done any wider reading, then do not panic. You do not need to start reading things just to say that you have done wider reading.

Try not to stress about having to learn and teach yourself a whole topic just so you can include it in your Veterinary Personal statement. Do not be unkind to yourself by stressing trying to force yourself to learn something you do not really enjoy (because also if it comes up at an interview this will show). The chances are, that if you have not done any wider reading, then you will likely have engaged with other academic hobbies and have academic achievements.

Talking about your wider reading at Veterinary Interviews

It is fair game for the interviewers to quiz you about anything you have written about. During your veterinary MMI / panel interview admissions officers may ask you about your insights and opinions relating to the books or journals named. If you choose to mention wider reading in your Veterinary Personal Statement, make sure you've actually researched it properly. Interviewers are not superhuman and clearly won't have read every piece of literature; despite this you never know what an interviewer has read or researched. Those interviewing you may have similar interests and be keen to engage in discussion on these topics.

When discussing your wider reading at your Veterinary interview our top tip is to stay calm and not panic. We reassure you that people often enjoy questions about their reading. Approach them as casual and intellectual discussions.

Top Tips for Writing About Your Veterinary Wider Reading

By taking on board our advice, you will be able to show that you have a genuine passion and interest in Veterinary. Being immersed into the world of Veterinary before you begin your training is key!

1. Don't list too many examples of wider reading

There is no set guidance for how many wider reading examples you should describe. Our general advice is to read as much as possible and make the most of all wider learning opportunities. Immerse yourself in super-curricular activities because you have a passion for science and are excited to study Veterinary medicine.

2. Include a variety of examples of wider reading

Engaging in super-curricular activities does not just mean reading books relating to Veterinary Science. Any form of wider reading about a topic of interest should be mentioned. Any form of wider reading shows that you are proactive, keen and intellectual.

3. Show don't tell

Aim not to just list what you have read in your Veterinary Personal Statement. Try to show excitement and passion. The following guidelines may give you some ideas of how to write about what you have read:
- State what it is that you found interesting.

- State what you've read (i.e. where it's from) – do not copy and paste the whole journal reference, but instead if you read something in a book (Dyce for example).
- State what about that topic that interests you.
- State how this is going to impact you as a future vet/ what you have learnt from this.

4. Keep it brief

Aim to write a sentence or two at most. Reflections on your wider reading should not make up the bulk of your Veterinary Personal Statement. Most of your personal statement should be paragraphs about your work experience and motivation for veterinary. Try not to lose focus. If you are very passionate about a particular topic you may get easily carried away writing about it adding excessive detail. Try to remember that the person reading the statement may know nothing about the topic you are talking about, you do not want to cause confusion. Show your enthusiasm for the topic, but in short bursts.

5. Structure your Veterinary Personal Statement appropriately

The best place to reference your wider reading is in the penultimate/ last paragraph of your Veterinary Personal Statement. Within this paragraph you should talk about your own achievements, hobbies etc, and relate them back to how this will make you a good vet.

Walkthrough Examples: Wider Reading Personal Statement

When writing about wider reading you have done in your Veterinary Personal Statement you want to consider your writing style. Below are examples of good and excellent reflections. Before you read our comments see if you can spot the difference between them yourself.

Veterinary PS: Example 1 – GOOD

'I particularly enjoyed reading about epigenetics from New Scientist magazine.'

This statement does have some merit. Name dropping "New Scientist" shows that the student has engaged with a reputable source. It indicates that the student has read higher level texts. However, this statement is very superficial. Admissions tutors may think that this student is simply 'fact-dropping'. The student could improve by being more specific as seen below.

Veterinary PS: Example 2- EXCELLENT

> 'My interest in epigenetics was sparked by my reading of New Scientist magazine, in particular, I find it fascinating how scientists are now using manipulation of epigenetics in veterinary to treat mammary cancers, in a process called epigenetic dysregulation. I look forward to learning more about this treatment in my time at vet school, and it has made me interested into where the future of veterinary medicine can be if this method is used to treat other diseases.'

This student is not just name dropping what they have read but they are discussing the content of their reading and contextualising it related to their application. Give it a go and try to link how your reading is relevant to being a vet.

Chapter 5: The ESAT - Cambridge University Admissions Test

What is the ESAT?
The Engineering and Science Admissions Test (or ESAT for short) is an exam which you have to take if you want to study the Natural Sciences, Veterinary Medicine or Chemical Engineering (via Natural Sciences) courses at the University of Cambridge. It is what is known as a 'pre-interview assessment', meaning that you sit the exam after you have submitted your UCAS application (and SAQ), but before you are (hopefully!) called to interview.

It is important to note that as of 2024, the ESAT has superceded the previous NSAA (Natural Sciences Admissions Assessment).

In this section, you'll read all the information on the ESAT exam, if you're applying or thinking about applying for any of these courses at Cambridge. So keep reading to get ahead of the game…

Why do I have to sit the ESAT exam?
You might be thinking, 'I'm already sitting GCSEs, Year 12 exams AND A-Levels, why do I need to take another test?!'. Well, according to the University of Cambridge, the test helps the ESAT admissions tutors decide if you will be the right fit for the Natural Sciences course, by assessing your level of knowledge of the relevant and required subject matter as well as your ability to apply that knowledge. Remember, Cambridge is not just looking for bright students, they are also looking for the right type of student, one who can apply the knowledge that they have to unfamiliar situations and someone who will thrive on these challenging courses.

Where and when do I take the ESAT exam?
You sit the ESAT at a test centre rather than at home, but for the vast majority of applicants the test centre is just your school, and other students will sit exams at the same time, for example, admissions tests for other Cambridge courses, as well as Oxford admissions tests and the UCAT for medicine.
The ESAT dates for 2024 are 15 and 16 October 2024.

What is the ESAT exam like?
The ESAT is split into 5 sections and depending on the course you are applying to, you will sit different sections. All candidates are required to sit the Mathematics 1 section. Candidates applying for Veterinary Science will then complete two additional sections from the list below:

- Biology
- Chemistry
- Physics
- Mathematics 2

All sections consist of 27 multiple-choice questions. You have 40 minutes for each ection, making the total length of the test 120 minutes.

Calculators are NOT allowed in any of the ESAT sections so mental maths skills are important!

What ESAT score should I be aiming for?

Unlike with your A-Level grades, for which there is an entry requirement (typically A*A*A), there is no target score for the ESAT, and it is not a pass or fail exam. The university provides some guidance on their website, stating that they don't expect candidates to be able to answer every question correctly in the allocated time. It is also important to note that no marks are deducted for incorrect answers so if you're not sure of an answer, it's better to guess than leave it blank!

It is important to remember that the ESAT is only one part of the admissions process, and is not taken as a pass-or-fail mark. The ESAT admissions tutors will take your mark in the exam into account along with all the other information you and your school submits, for example, your grades so far, your personal statement, your references from teachers and your interview performance. This means that although it's important to try your best, the ESAT is not the be-all and end-all of your admission to Cambridge, so try to keep calm, practise the ESAT practice papers, and just be as prepared as you can.

ESAT Sections and Specifications

The specifications for the ESAT sections are largely similar to a GCSE syllabus, with Mathematics 2 being more aligned with the A-Level syllabus. All questions are multiple-choice which gives you a significant advantage if you are unsure. You can employ exam techniques such a ruling out answers to minimise your options. Below is a list of the main specification points for each section. Please note that each specification point is further broken down into expectations. If you want to know more about the specification, you can visit the official website at https://esat-tmua.ac.uk/. The website also has example papers and timed tests for you to practise before the exam.

Mathematics 1

All candidates are required to take Mathematics 1, despite the course you are applying to. You are NOT allowed to use a calculator in any part of the exam so be sure to practise your mental maths! Here are the main specification points for this section.

M1 - Units	M5 - Geometry
M2 - Number	M6 - Statistics
M3 - Ration & Proportion	M7 - Probability
M4 - Algebra	

Mathematics 2

Although the questions in this section are harder than the ones in Mathematics 1, you are still NOT allowed a calculator. While this may seem daunting, it does mean that the questions will have been purposely set in order for you to do calculations in your head or use methods such as rounding and elimination to find the right answer. Her are the main specification points for this section.

MM1 - Algebra & Functions	MM5 - Exponentials & Logarithms
MM2 - Sequences & Series	MM6 - Differentiation
MM3 - Coordinate Geometry	MM7 - Integration
MM4 - Trigonometry	MM8 - Graphs of Functions

Physics

The specification points largely follow the GCSE syllabus with some A-Level content. You may also be required to answer some calculation questions in Physics.

P1 - Electricity	P5 - Matter
P2 - Magnetism	P6 - Waves
P3 - Mechanics	P7 - Radioactivity
P4 - Thermal Physics	

Biology

If you are taking the Biology section of the ESAT, don't be put off by the increased number of specification points. Visit the official website to see the specification broken down so you are aware of what you should revise.

B1 - Cells	B5 - DNA
B2 - Movement Across Membranes	B6 - Gene Technologies
B3 - Cell Division & Sex determination	B7 - Variation
B4 - Inheritance	B8 - Enzymes
B9 - Animal Physiology	B10 - Ecosystems
B11 - Plant Physiology	

Chemistry

As with the Biology section, don't be put off by the number of specification points. If you feel that Chemistry is a strong subject of yours, then be confident in your abilities. You may be asked calculation questions so remember that you cannot use a calculator!

C1 - Atomic Structure	C10 - Rates of Reaction
C2 - The Periodic Table	C11 - Energetics
C3 - Chemical Reactions, Formulae & Equations	C12 - Electrolysis
C4 - Quantitative Chemistry	C13 - Carbon/Organic Chemistry
C5 - Oxidation, Reduction, & Redox	C14 - Metals
C6 - Chemical Bonding, Structure & Properties	C15 - Kinetic/Particle Theory
C7 - Group Chemistry	C16 - Chemical Tests
C8 - Separation Techniques	C17 Air & Water
C9 - Acids, Bases & Salts	

Timing

One of the things candidates struggle with the most in any exam, but especially a multiple-choice exam, is TIMING. I'm sorry to say that the ESAT is no exception. You will have 40 minutes to complete each section, so that means 40 minutes for 27 questions. That works out to be (opportunity for mental arithmetic practice here!) 1 minute 30 seconds (!!) per question. This is NOT a lot of time!

Now, I'm not telling you this to stress you out (that's the last thing we want) but just so that you are prepared. The best way to deal with this is simply to practise ESAT practice questions under timed conditions, as these will not be of a similar format to questions you have done before, say in your GCSEs or Year 12 exams.

What you need to know

The ESAT website very helpfully provides a specification which tells you everything you need to know and understand for the exam, broken down by section.

You should also make sure you are familiar and comfortable with the use of SI units (standard units for scientific quantities), as well as how different SI units are linked and inter converted. Candidates should also be happy with the use of SI prefixes, such as milli- or kilo-, and what these mean, in addition to the use of negative indices, like ms-1 instead of m/s. There is a list of the SI prefixes expected contained in the specification, but it is from giga- down to nano-.

Top Tips for the ESAT Exam

1. Start preparing well in advance
This sounds obvious, but you'd be surprised at how quickly the test will come around once you start with the chaos of year 13! The exam is usually taken in early November, so I would recommend starting your ESAT preparations in August since you will have A-Level work to focus on once school or college starts back in September.

2. Read through the specification thoroughly
The ESAT website provides a specification containing a list of all the content you are required to know, understand and could be tested on. This is important because remember that not every student will have taken the same exams up to this point (for example different countries around the world have different qualifications) and not every school (even within the UK) will have taught the same A-Level (or equivalent) content up to the point of taking the exam.

This means you can't assume that you will have covered everything on the exam, however, since it is mostly based on applying GCSE content in ways you are unfamiliar with, you will most likely not have to learn too many new things.

3. Have a go at as many ESAT practice questions as possible
I cannot stress enough how important this is! The style of questions asked on the ESAT will be unfamiliar to you, so the absolute best way to be as prepared as possible is to practise using ESAT sample questions. This is quite tricky as the ESAT is a new exam from 2024 so past papers will not be available. However, they will be similar in style to the previous NSAA test so it is a good idea to practise NSAA past papers as well.

4. Make sure you're registered by your school well in advance of the test
It is your responsibility to ensure that:
- Your school is a registered test centre (if it is not, your school can apply to become a test centre (there is a deadline for this which is usually the end of September) or you can find a different test centre near you)
- You are registered for the test (you will need your UCAS number for this)
- You have your candidate number, which is also your proof of registration

All of these things can be done by speaking to the exams officer at your school or college, and more information about registration can be found on the admissions testing website.

5. Practice under timed conditions
Multiple-choice tests are notoriously difficult when it comes to timing, and the ESAT is no exception. You don't have very much time per question (only 1.5 minutes).
This means that practising some ESAT sample questions under timed conditions is really good practice to get a feel of the pace that you're going to have to work at to answer as

many questions as possible. I wouldn't recommend doing all of your revision under timed conditions as this could be a little stressful, but certainly work up to it once you feel that you have an idea of the style of the questions.

6. Practise your mental arithmetic
Every candidate is required to complete the Mathematics 1 section and this is done without a calculator, as are the other sections! This means any and all calculations will need to be done in your head (but you will of course have a pencil and paper too so it's not completely mental maths!). A lot of students struggle with this so I would definitely recommend practising extra mental maths as part of your ESAT revision if you think this might be a weak point for you.

7. Don't stress!
Remember that the ESAT is not a pass or fail exam, and admissions tutors will not completely disregard your application if you don't do as well on the day as you could have done. The ESAT test is only one part of your application to Cambridge and will be looked at alongside all of your other work, such as exam grades (or teacher assessed grades), predicted grades, personal statement, SAQ and references from teachers. There is no ESAT minimum score' that you need to get, so all you can do is practise ESAT practice questions, remain as calm as possible on the day and try your best!

VETERINARY LIVE MMI CIRCUIT

- ✓ Written by real MMI examiners, and trusted by schools

- ✓ Perform 10 live MMI stations yourself, completing a full circuit, and then pair up to observe an additional 10 stations!

- ✓ Experience a wide range of stations, covering role plays, veterinary ethics, hot topics, work experience, and more

Book Your Place Today!

Find out more at https://www.medicmind.co.uk/vet-school-mmi-circuit/ or scan the QR code below

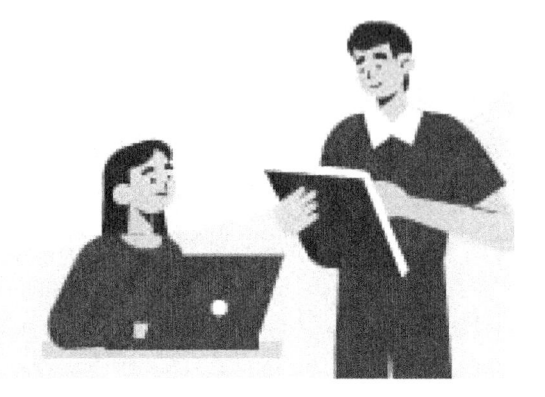

VETERINARY INTERVIEW ONLINE COURSE

- [✓] 100+ tutorials, and 100+ MMI stations, designed by our Dentistry interview experts

- [✓] Learn how to answer questions on motivation for Dentistry, personal skills, work experience, hot topics, and more

- [✓] A range of packages available, including a live day of teaching and 1:1 tutoring

Buy Now!

Find out more at https://www.medicmind.co.uk/veterinary-medicine-interview-course/ or scan the QR code below

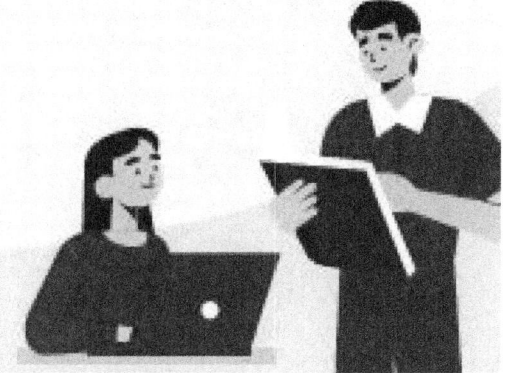

1:1 VET INTERVIEW TUTORING

✓ Delivered by current Dentistry students, who excelled in the interview themselves

✓ A personalised 1:1 approach, tailored to your unique needs

✓ An overall 93.4% success rate, with students improving their performance by an average of 57.3%

Book your FREE consultation now

For more information, visit https://www.medicmind.co.uk/vet-interview-tutors/ or scan the QR code below

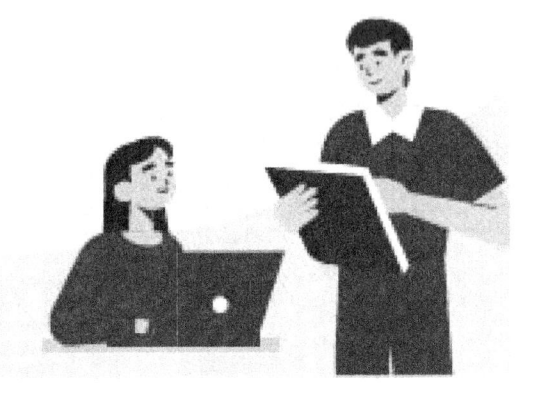

Chapter 6: Veterinary Interview

Types of Veterinary Interview

Interview structure
The style of interview varies considerably between vet schools. Many vet schools now use multiple mini interviews (MMIs), which involve a series of individually assessed stations testing a variety of skills. However, some universities still use traditional panel interviews which take on a more conversational format. You should identify the interview structure each vet school you have applied to uses, so that you can tailor your preparation accordingly. Please bear in mind that universities have the right to change interview styles and structures between years, so information regarding previous application cycles may not be applicable to you. Ensure you read all communication directly from the vet school about your interview very carefully to ensure you know what to expect on the day.

Multiple Mini Interviews (MMIs)
Also colloquially known as MMIs, multiple mixed interviews offer a 'speed-dating' approach with your interviewer. Typically, there are around 5 MMI stations in an MMI interview. These will be held one after the other with each station assessing different skills and displaying different formats. For example, one MMI station might test your anatomy knowledge by presenting you with two diagrams, cadavers or real-life skeletons! where you may need to compare and explain the skeletal anatomy of a horse vs a dog. However, your MMI station after this may test your understanding of ethics by presenting you with an ethical dilemma and asking how you would respond. Along with these skills and knowledge based stations, you will likely also be asked more traditional interview questions such as why you want to study Veterinary Medicine or why you wish to study at that particular university.

Some universities will offer a short section of reading time (usually 1 minute) prior to each station in order to prepare your answer, particularly if the station is based on a sample of a reading material or a diagram that you need to review and answer questions on. For those universities which do not offer this, you should start preparing your answer on pen and paper if available as the interviewer is running you through the question. Preparing your answer this way allows for a concise and well-thought out response. One great advantage of the MMI interview system is how performance and scores in each interview is collected and reviewed. Performed poorly in your team work station? Do not stress and move on!

The best approach to the MMI is to take each station like it is your first - do not get hung up on mistakes previously made as your interviewer for station 5 will never ever know that you did not know how to label the hind limb skeleton in station 3. Keep calm and focus on the next station.

The vet schools currently adopting this MMI system include:
- Edinburgh
- Harper-Keele
- Liverpool
- Surrey
- RVC

Panel interviews

The most traditional form of interview is made up of multiple interviewers asking a series of questions and the entire interview can range from 20-40 minutes long. The number of people on the panel ranges from 2-3 and can be a good mix of personnel. This may include older vet students on the course, professors at the university, and clinical vets themselves. Unlike MMIs, panel interviews feel less time pressured, as they will feel very conversational and you can refer back to comments made in previous questions to help you answer the next one. This is why some students prefer a panel interview, as you can build on your answers with each question that is asked and potentially feel more focused and therefore more calm.

Mixed interviews

Due to there being no requirement to sit the UCAT for the vet school application, mixed interviews are common when reviewing vet school applications. After submitting your personal statement, some UK vet schools (currently Surrey and Nottingham) will send out a Situational Judgement Test (SJT). As well as being done pre-interview, situational judgement assessments may be done at the beginning of a panel interview. It is important to know that this is just another way vet schools assess students to be able to pick the best out of the many. A situational judgement assessment simply assesses how you will respond and subsequently act as a vet.

Essentially, the SJT puts you in different scenarios and assesses you on how you act and deal with the situation at hand. Although not all the scenarios will be related to Veterinary Medicine, you should keep in mind that your answer should follow the basic ethics and values of a vet.

For example, a non-related vet SJT question could be 'You are sitting an exam and notice a friend sitting beside you is looking over at your answers and copying you… what do you do?'

With this type of scenario-based question, you may be presented with a list of possible responses you could take. For example:

- I would do nothing as it is none of my business if someone cheats
- I would immediately tell the teacher that the student is copying me
- I would wait till the end of the exam and tell the head teacher that they were copying me

- I would wait until after the exam to talk to the student, to inform them that copying is cheating and they should tell the teacher about the situation.

You are then asked to rank these in order of most to least appropriate, and your order will be assessed on the basis of what is actually deemed appropriate.

What To Wear To A Vet School Interview

Where to start?
Let's start with you receiving your veterinary interview invite! This is a great achievement! Congratulations! The veterinary interview process is a competitive one and you've made it to the next stage. Woohoo!

Once all of the excitement is out of the way and the reality of your interview kicks in, the vet school interview can suddenly seem quite daunting. This is your opportunity to shine and you want everything to be perfect. So naturally this leads you on to wonder about what to wear to a vet interview.

A fashion show?
Ball gowns and black tuxedos away, this is not a catwalk! The interview isn't about who can afford the most expensive suit from London or a glittery dress from New York. The interview isn't about who looks the most glamorous and dazzling. Save your high heels for a better occasion. There is no need to go and spend a fortune, most people already have something suitable.

What to wear to a vet school interview: an interviewer's perspective
The interviewers want to get to know you better. The purpose of the interview is to see how you think logically and to get a sense of what kind of person you are, so if you're kind, empathetic and understanding. The dress code will always be smart or smart casual for an interview and your clothing can be a great way to show your personality. I'm not saying to wear a hoodie because you enjoy lounging around on a lazy Sunday morning, but I'm saying it's okay to show who you are.

What to wear to a vet interview: What I would recommend
I personally wore a brown leather pair of loafers, with a smart pair of black jeans (without rips- I don't like cold knees!) and a blue blouse, finishing this with a cream cardigan. I didn't own a suit or similar, so I used what I had. This was a smart casual look that I felt comfortable in, even if I do say so myself!

I'm very much not the type of person to wear a suit and I wanted to show that I was a little different, without being too out there. I made this look personal to me, by wearing my favourite watch and a locket necklace, but obviously this is optional.
As long as you look smart, the interviewers won't notice what you are wearing- there are much more important things to consider!!

For guys, I would recommend a smart pair of trousers, definitely with a shirt, and perhaps a classy jumper to finish. Avoid trainers at all costs; leather shoes might be a better alternative. Ties are optional, some people like them, some people hate them, so go with what you feel comfortable in.

What to wear to a vet school interview: What everyone else wears

Typically, guys tend to wear suits. There is no need for a waistcoat or the really posh accessories. If I'm honest, I doubt that the interviewer's would even notice! Navy and black suits with leather shoes are the most popular and nearly all of the men wear shirts.

For the girls, there is a little more flexibility. Some girls tend to go for the suit option and some tend to go for a blouse with smart trousers. Equally, some girls wear dresses and skirts, though this is a little less common.

What to wear to a vet interview: Let's be practical

The universities enjoy the opportunity to show off their campuses and try and attract the potential new students. Quite often this means walking outside following a student ambassador. Some of the vet schools up north in the UK can be pretty chilly and windy! You'd show yourself to be a better candidate if you listen to the student ambassador, rather than standing there moaning about the weather conditions. Make sure that your footwear is suitable for walking and is not going to give you blisters!

What to wear to a vet school interview: Do's and Don'ts

Do:
- Dress smart or smart casually, depending on the university requests
- Bring a jacket, preferably rain proof, and something to keep warm
- Do show your personal style, while remaining smart casual.

Don't:
- Wear high heels and other uncomfortable shoes for walking
- Avoid dresses or skirts that are likely to blow up in the wind
- Spend a fortune on a designer outfit

On the day of the interview

This day can be stressful enough, without the need to maintain make-up or deal with tricky outfits. The interviewers want to get to know you and you can show them your best side in something comfortable and smart. The interview day really isn't a fashion show, so please don't panic too much about this!!

The best thing that you can wear is your smile. This shows the interviewers the type of person that you are and how you can remain positive under pressure. Your smile is invaluable!

How to Prepare for a Vet School Interview

Although this is a time to get excited, it's also a great opportunity to pick up some handy interview tips. Preparation is key to smashing your vet school interview and showing your vet school why you deserve a place. Do keep reading, I'd love to share my tips with you for how to prepare for a vet school interview.

What might the interviewers ask?

Let's just recap on what sort of question categories that you could be asked at your interview;
- Ethics
- Role Play
- Anatomy
- Topical Issues
- Work Experience

What are the answers to the questions?

Okay, so I know what they might ask me about, but the topics are so broad, I hear you say! And oh yes they are! But the big big similarity between the topics is what? YOU! It is you that answers the questions and in doing this you show the university how you can think logically and apply your knowledge. Yes, of course your answers are important, but how you get to your answers is so much more than about being right or wrong.

Top tips on how to prepare for a vet school interview

1. Explain your reasoning

The whole point of the interview is for the university to see how you think- so show them! The interviewers will ask you questions to understand how you come to your conclusions, how you can apply your knowledge and how you can justify your answers. If you explain every decision that you make, the examiner can sit back in their chair and go "Yes, yes yes! Give this student an offer!"

Let's have a look at an example showing how you can achieve this;
If the interviewer asks what the organ is that they are showing you, you could respond in two ways.

   a. *"The organ is the liver."*

This answers the examiner's question but doesn't expand on why. The examiner will then have to ask your more questions to understand why you think in this way.

    b. *"The organ is the liver because it is dark in colour, has a smooth surface with some rounded edges. I can see that this structure also has flappy bits, which might be the liver lobes."*

This shows the examiner your logic- great! This also puts you in control of the conversation, meaning that you give answers before they have been asked and means that you can guide the conversation towards things that you are comfortable to talk about.

2. Learn the detail of your personal statement

This is such a good detail to include in your plan of how to prepare for a vet school interview. The vet school wants to know what you know, not what you don't! You're not expected to be a vet before vet school! You have provided each university with a copy of your personal statement, and this gives them a little insight into what you have learned from your experiences so far. To help you out, the examiners like to ask questions on what you have learned, to give you the best shot at answering them confidently.

Here's an example showing how you can wow the examiner;
If the examiner asks you about your time that you spent in a vet clinic you could say;

    a. *"I spent lots of time watching the vets give animals vaccinations."*

This is something that most people do and doesn't show that you have learned anything from your experience. This also doesn't make you sound that interesting. The examiner has to ask you another question to try and draw more answers out of you.

    b. *"I spent lots of time watching puppies have their first vaccinations. I know that one disease puppies are vaccinated against is Canine Parvovirus Disease. I think that this causes the puppies to vomit and have severe bloody diarrhoea if they get infected. The puppies are vaccinated at 8 and 12 weeks old."*

This answer shows that you have researched further into what you have seen. A great way to get your veterinary offer is to show that you are keen and want to learn!

3. Smile!

This sounds so obvious, but smiling ticks a box that the interviewers are looking for. Academic knowledge and correct answers are great, but you will need so much more than this to become a good vet. The interviewer's want to see how you cope when put under pressure. Interview days are stressful for anyone, so take this as an opportunity to show how well you can do. Smiling shows the examiner that you are enjoying what you are talking about and you are keen, but what else? It shows that you are not worried about the pressure (even though you might be a little nervous!) and that you are determined to enjoy the interview. These are great qualities of a future vet!

4. Prepare for the obvious!

If you're applying to vet school, the university will want to know why! They want to know what makes you want to be a vet and what makes you want to go to that specific university. Linking this with your experience and any extra research that you have done will make you stand out amongst the crowd.

5. Stay up to date on key veterinary issues

There will always be so many topical issues in veterinary medicine. These range from the shortage of vets to the breeding of brachycephalic dogs. If you're aware of some of these problems and would feel comfortable to talk about them, the interviewers will recognise how keen you are. They'll love it! And you never know, you might learn something new too. The Vet Record is a great online resource for this.

6. Think about the question carefully

Each question that you are asked is designed to help the university to get to know you better. If you can identify what the university wants to know, you get the opportunity to tick their box and show them that they need you in their vet school. Make them desperate to have you!

7. Show your best self in the group task

The whole point of a group task is to identify how well you work with others, so show them! This type of station tests your communication skills with the other applicants.

One great way to wow the interviewers is to start by introducing yourself to the group and asking everyone else to introduce themselves. Using everyone's names shows how attentive you are and how you want to work as a group to get to the solution.

8. Reflect on your previous experiences

Work experience is a huge part of getting into vet school and the interviewers love to ask you about it. If you can learn a case that you saw in practice- great! You could take this one step further by reflecting on what you have seen and discussing what did and didn't go well. This shows that you have engaged with your experiences and how you want to improve- a very very important quality.

9. Dress appropriately

The interview isn't a fashion show! There is definitely no need for a new ball gown! You want to show yourself professionally, but it's okay to show a bit of your style too! Avoid the hoodies and trainers, go for something on the smart-casual to smart spectrum. Each university normally advises students what to wear, so go with that.

10. Practise, practise and practise!

You really can't do enough of this. Most people worry about having a blank and not knowing what to say. This is completely understandable and one way to get rid of those nerves is to go through some example questions. Once you get into the swing of things, you should find yourself relaxing and opening up.

And so…

Interview days are daunting for everyone. Knowing how to prepare for the vet school interview sets you one step ahead of everyone else. So remember: explain your reasoning, learn the details of your personal statement, and smile! It's up to you to show the universities that you should get a place. Go and get it!

In need of more advice? The Association of Veterinary Students provides a great guide on getting into vet school.

TOP Vet Interview Questions You Should Be Prepared To Answer

Veterinary medicine is such a competitive process so receiving an invitation to the vet school interview is something to be proud of! Maybe now you are wondering what might happen at your veterinary medicine interview? Or how you should prepare to answer the top veterinary medicine interview questions? Great decision; you're already on track to smashing your vet school interview.

Interview questions for vet school understandably cause lots of nerves in students for different reasons. The most important thing to remember is that vet interview questions really aren't scary! I like to think of them as an informal chat, rather than an intense interrogation. Think of this as an opportunity to show each vet school who you are and why you deserve a place on their course. Show your enthusiasm and smile, your passion and motivation.

What are the key vet interview questions that you're likely to be asked, I hear you say. Each university has a preference on the type of veterinary medicine interview questions that they like to ask, but the overall MMI station themes are:

- Ethics
- Role Play
- Anatomy
- Topical Issues
- Work Experience

The list of interview questions for vet school could go on and on and on! The Association of Veterinary Students gives some really nice examples of specific questions that you might be asked.

There are thousands of veterinary medicine interview questions that you could be asked, so instead of thinking about the textbook answer for each possibility, have a think about this: What do the interviewer's want to see from me? What will make the vet school fall in love with me? And the answer to that lies in the question... YOU!

What the examiners are really looking for is to get to know you. To know how you think, to know how you prioritise, to know how you work under pressure. Everything that goes at the interview helps them to get to know you as a person, and the MMI stations are a great way of doing this!

Let's have a little look at the type of vet interview questions and how you can make the vet school desperate to give you an offer.

Ethics

Ethical stations focus on the challenges that a vet might experience in their day-to-day life. Typical interview questions for vet school focus on euthanasia, financial barriers to treatment and knowing how to deal with tricky clients. Again, the questions for this topic could go on and on and on. In need of an easy fool-proof approach? We've got you sorted!

Vet school interview tips for ethics stations

The key to tackling ethical situations is to think about everyone that is affected by the decision made, and when I say everyone, I mean everyone! Think about the owner, the vet, the pet, the consumer, the farmer, the finances, the other staff, the public, the family, other animals- if you can name it, you can talk about it! Showing a wider understanding of who our decisions can affect and why we may or may not choose to act in the way that we do will have you onto a winner.

Role-Play

Understandably, lots of applicants are slightly nervous about this station. The myths surrounding scary actors that shout and cry just aren't true. The main purpose of this station is to see how you can think about a problem and come up with multiple solutions. Along the way, the actors may challenge you and encourage you to expand your thinking. This is a good sign, such a good sign! By challenging you, the actors are testing you under pressure. They want to see how you respond and can change your thinking, whilst showing a genuine display of empathy and emotion. And if the situation starts to get tricky, this is a great thing!

Vet school interview tips for role play stations

You have been given the opportunity to show yourself off under pressure. Take this opportunity to show how confident you are and show the actors that you do deserve a place on the vet course. Take these stations seriously by getting into character and responding how you imagine a real vet would.

Anatomy

Some universities like to throw in an anatomy station to test you. This is likely to have been something covered by your A-Level Biology course or it could be something that you have little knowledge about.

Revising the basic structure of each organ in the body and how this relates to its function will help you massively. It can also be helpful to look at online X-rays of dogs and cats to try identify simple structures e.g a heart.

An important part of this station is to expect to be challenged. Sometimes this may be incorporated into a maths question, to push you a bit further.

Vet school interview tips for anatomy stations
Please don't eat an entire degree textbook in the hope to become an anatomist before vet school! What the interviewer's really want to see here is how you think and come up with new ideas. Accept this as an opportunity to learn.

Nobody expects you to be a vet before vet school! And remember, this station also tests how you respond to pressure. The interviewer will ask you questions until you get to something that you don't know. They are looking to push you and see how you respond.

Lots of students are worried that they will blank and panic. The best way to tackle that on this vet interview station is to talk about what you do know, think about how you can relate that to this scenario, and ask the interviewer to explain the answer if you get it wrong. This shows that you are keen!

Topical Issues
The vet interview question surrounding topical issues doesn't require a comprehensive, essay-worthy response, but an overview of some of the topical issues relating to veterinary. Focusing on the advantages and disadvantages of all possible options will really help you to secure your offer.

Vet school interview tips for topical issues stations
Adding your opinion once you have weighed up the advantages and disadvantages adds a nice touch to your answer. Common issues spoken about would be the breeding of brachycephalic dogs, veganism and the increase in pet ownership during the COVID 19 pandemic. Prior research will show that you are keen, feel free to mention news articles and statistics you may have come across, but be careful to avoid biased sources. Try to have a balanced approach throughout your response before coming to a justified conclusion.

Work Experience
This is the time for you to shine! Since YOU are being asked the interview questions for vet school, your response must be specific to YOU! Making a diary of all of your work experiences will help you massively in this type of station.

Vet school interview tips for work experience stations
My biggest bit of advice would be to pick a case in veterinary practice that you have seen and to learn it as best as you can. It doesn't have to be an elaborate or life-threatening case, but something that you have found interesting. Learning about the clinical signs, the diagnostic tests or imaging, the diagnosis itself and the treatment plan will stand you in good stead. But do remember, your work experience must be specific to you.

Want more common questions?

Example veterinary medicine interview questions are a great way to get you on your way to receiving your offer. Here are some examples for you to get stuck into…

1. Why do you want to do veterinary medicine?
2. What aspect of animal welfare attracts you to veterinary medicine?
3. What steps have you taken to try to find out whether you really do want to become a vet?
4. Why should we give you a place?
5. What attributes do you have that will make you a good vet?
6. Could you think of a situation where your communication skills made a difference to the outcome of a situation?
7. Give an example where you have played an effective role as a team member.
8. What makes you a good team leader?
9. Veterinary medicine requires a great deal of independent study and organisation. How will you manage it?
10. Give an example of a situation where you have made a mistake and how you reacted
11. Studying for veterinary medicine is a long and stressful process. What makes you think that you can cope with it?
12. You will probably have got high marks throughout school. On this vet course, most marks are awarded as 'satisfactory' or not. How will you feel about seeing 'average' in this new situation?
13. What did you learn from your work experience?
14. How did your work experience change your view of veterinary medicine?
15. What are the challenges of being a vet?
16. Do you believe that euthanasia should be allowed?
17. How are farm animals treated differently to pet animals?
18. Is it right to cull farm animals that have a slower productivity? (e.g. laying hens that don't lay eggs anymore)
19. What do you know about the badger cull in preventing TB?
20. How can vets help prevent the problems associated with brachycephalic breeds?

Veterinary Interview Scenarios & MMI Stations

Motivation for Veterinary Medicine

Question 1
What do you wish to achieve in your career in veterinary medicine, aside from clinical practice?

Example 1
"I would like to focus my studies and thus my career on small animal surgery and the hopes of one day owning and running my own first opinion practice. While I was on my work experience placement, I got to shadow the practice owner and ask him about the qualities it takes to run a small animal veterinary clinic. Therefore, when I become a small animal surgeon, I look forward to working my way up to opening a private practice and having a more of a management role as well"

Feedback
This is a poor answer. While the student attempts to reflect on their work experience, they do so superficially and only identify opportunities in the management sector of veterinary medicine. This comes across as money motivated and shows a lack of insight into management opportunities. Furthermore, there are no links to the candidate's own skills to evidence their career motivations.

Example 2
"I hope to become involved in academic research alongside my clinical career. During my work experience placement at a small animal practice, I met a owner who was consenting for their pet (the patient) to take part in a clinical trial due to their condition, which highlighted to me the important interaction of biomedical research and patient care. While researching your veterinary school, I was particularly excited by the opportunity to take an intercalated research year during the degree as this would explore my research interests further and gain valuable experience."

Feedback
This is a good answer. The student identifies a suitable area of non-clinical practice and demonstrates an understanding of why research is important. The student also shows initiative by having plans to become involved in research early in their career. Notably, the candidate mentions opportunities to do so at the vet school in question which echoes a sense of commitment to researching potential career pathways and opportunities. This will be well received by interviewers.

Work Experience

Question 1
What are the skills required by a first opinion small animal vet?

"A vet working in a small animal clinic needs to be knowledgeable and up-to-date in the management of conditions spanning every medical speciality. Additionally, many soft-skills are required for good clinical practice including, open mindedness, time efficiency and the ability to multitask.

During my work experience in this field I particularly noticed the need for a vet to possess strong communication skills. Vets will see a wide variety of patients and clients who have a range of communication needs. The owner is involved, as well as the patient who can't even talk! Communication between the vet and the owner is vital and they need to be as clear as possible so the owner understands what is going on with their pet. A vet needs to be in-tune with and be able to adapt to these varying needs of the human-animal bond within a short timeframe. For example, I recall the vet seeing a border collie patient whose owner trains dogs for the cruft competitions and then in the next appointment just 10 minutes later, they had to communicate to a first time owner of a shih tzu puppy."

Explanation
This question is an excellent opportunity to discuss observations you made during your work experience. There are a vast number of skills you could mention, but try to pick a handful to discuss in depth with support from scenarios in your work experience. An excellent answer would reflect on these experiences and provide examples where they also demonstrate the skill in question.

Question 2
How do small animal practices prioritise patients?

"As a small animal first opinion vet works under time pressure, it is critical that patients who are more seriously unwell are given priority. When I undertook a work experience placement at my local veterinary practice, patients' owners were initially booked for short telephone consultations. The receptionist and sometimes the vet nurse used these telephone calls to assess the severity of symptoms and determine which patients needed to be seen in-person that day.

In some cases the vet surgeon was confident enough to diagnose over the phone, which had the benefit of saving the patient time to come into the clinic.

While the telephone triage system can save time, I recall a scenario where a client became upset with the system as they felt that they had not been properly assessed due to their cat who was unwell not being physically examined.

This made me consider the patient and client perspective due to the human-animal bond and how a patient being triaged as non-urgent could be interpreted to the client as receiving a lower standard of care. Some vet practices have opted to use alternative triaging systems for this, among other reasons."

Explanation
This question is looking for candidates to have considered the important task of *triage*, which refers to the process of deciding which order patients should be seen in. The student is able to reflect on their work experience to describe the prioritisation process they observed, while also having an appreciation of positive and negative aspects of the system.

Question 3
How long did each appointment last for? Did you feel this was an appropriate appointment length?

"Each first opinion vet appointment is typically just 10 minutes long as standard. I found that for some patients this was sufficient to explore their symptoms and recommend a management plan. However, for some patients with more complex, or multiple, issues the 10 minute time slot was restrictive to the amount of depth that could be explored.

For example, I can recall a particular patient, a 4-year old cat, at her appointment regarding constant itching. The vet skilfully fully explored her symptoms and prescribed a treatment within the appointment slot, but just as the consultation was ending the owner wanted to tell the vet her cat had also been suffering from diarrhoea and wanted to discuss this too. This demonstrates how difficult having such tight time limits can be, as time efficiency must be balanced with showing you care and have time for the patient without them feeling rushed."

Explanation
Vet first opinion appointment times are often difficult to stick to, but 10 minutes is standard across the UK. Owners frequently complain about being called later than their appointment time due to previous appointments over-running which can strain the relationship between vet and client before the appointment has even begun.

This question is looking for a student to understand the strain of appointment length on vets and to demonstrate some insight into the challenges this poses for veterinarians.

Question 4
What is the role and importance of the vet receptionist?

"I was lucky enough to spend an afternoon with the reception team while on my work experience placement in a small animal first opinion practice.

I observed the receptionists booking appointments, dealing with client requests and liaising with the veterinarians and nurses when needed. Overall, my time with the reception staff demonstrated the importance of organisation within veterinary healthcare systems, as without the work performed by reception staff the whole system would cease to function."

Explanation
By asking this question, an interviewer is making sure candidates have an understanding and appreciation for the critical work other members of the healthcare team, including non-clinical staff, perform to improve patient care.

Question 5
What are the skills required by a first opinion small animal vet?

"A vet working in a small animal clinic needs to be knowledgeable and up-to-date in the management of conditions spanning every medical speciality. Additionally, many soft-skills are required for good clinical practice including, open mindedness, time efficiency and the ability to multitask.

During my work experience in this field I particularly noticed the need for a vet to possess strong communication skills. Vets will see a wide variety of patients and clients who have a range of communication needs. The owner is involved, as well as the patient who can't even talk! Communication between the vet and the owner is vital and they need to be as clear as possible so the owner understands what is going on with their pet. A vet needs to be in-tune with and be able to adapt to these varying needs of the human-animal bond within a short timeframe.

For example, I recall the vet seeing a border collie patient whose owner trains dogs for the cruft competitions and then in the next appointment just 10 minutes later, they had to communicate to a first time owner of a shih tzu puppy."

Explanation
This question is an excellent opportunity to discuss observations you made during your work experience. There are a vast number of skills you could mention, but try to pick a handful to discuss in depth with support from scenarios in your work experience. An excellent answer would reflect on these experiences and provide examples where they also demonstrate the skill in question.

Question 6
Can you tell me about a surgery you have seen?

"During my work experience at my local veterinary clinic, I was lucky enough to witness a female dog being spayed which the vet surgeon later told me the correct term to be an ovariohysterectomy.

The vet nurse, who I got to witness prep the surgery by keeping everything hygienic to avoid unwanted bacterial transmission, told me how this type of surgery was becoming less popular than it was 20 years ago. The veterinary surgeon then went on to tell me the importance of neutering as a form of preventive medicine. Female dogs can develop an infection called pyometra which results in the need for emergency surgery as it can cause death if untreated. As I learnt this only occurs in dogs without having an ovariohysterectomy surgery, it highlighted to me how preventive medicine for patients is in my opinion in their best interest to stop sickness before it starts."

Explanation
The key aspect of this question is to recognise the reasoning behind certain surgeries. The student goes on to talk about preventive medicine which is important in deciding whether surgery is appropriate or not in certain cases. Overall this is an excellent answer.

Question 7
What skills does a good vet surgeon have?

"Small animal vet surgeons are required to be knowledgeable, work in a team and have good communication skills. In addition, due to the practical nature of their job, a surgeon must have incredible manual dexterity skills.

During my work experience, I was amazed by how small some of the anatomical structures operated on were. This reinforced the importance of precision to a surgeon's work.

I was given the opportunity to observe a cyst removal during my work experience. Unfortunately, there were complications as the patient began to bleed. This scenario, while initially startling to me, demonstrated how a vet surgeon's ability to maintain composure in difficult situations is critical. I noticed how the vet demeanour often sets the tone of the room, which was particularly key in this case as the patient was awake."

Explanation
Different types of vets draw on different skill sets and this question is asking candidate's to reflect on their observations of surgeons to discuss the skills particularly relevant to their job. An excellent candidate would suggest ways in which they have, or plan to, develop these same skills.

Question 8
Have you read an article or interesting news topic relating to surgery?

"I have recently read an article from the vet times regarding a life threatening incident due to something so common and once thought harmless.

An owner has been playing with her dog in the park and had thrown her a stick, once at home and the next day the dog's owner had noticed her dog was fatigued and had blood in her vomit. Once at the vets, it was discovered that the stick had nipped a vital blood vessel in the back of the dog's throat. In order to locate such an intricate blood vessel cut, a team of soft tissue specialists used a video endoscope to identify the entry site of the wound in order to stop excessive bleeding. This was similar to a case I got to see during my work experience where the sharp wood of a stick got caught in a dog's soft padding on their paw. However, as it was an external injury, no intricate entering of the cavity was needed to discover the site of the injury.

<u>Explanation</u>
By showing evidence of further reading around topics relevant to work experience, the candidate is showing they are genuinely interested in veterinary medicine and have the drive to learn more. Similarly a vet student may be expected to use their evenings to read up on conditions they have seen on placement that day. If you are asked a question like this, expect to be asked follow-up questions about your opinions. Consequently, never pretend to have read something you have not!

Personal Qualities & Skills

Question 1

Give three adjectives that best describe you.

"The first adjective I would use to describe myself is organised. Alongside studying for my A-Level exams, I have taken on multiple additional responsibilities such as Head of the animal welfare society over the past year. This required substantial organisation, to ensure smooth running of all society activities, alongside meeting academic deadlines and maintaining grades. Developing strong organisation skills is important for a career as a veterinarian, where prioritisation of tasks and patients is key. I would also describe myself using the adjectives leader and empathetic."

<u>Feedback</u>
This question invites candidates to discuss three skills of their choice. You may not have time to fully explore each skill and link it back to veterinary medicine. This answer opts to discuss organisation in full, and simply mentions leadership and empathy without discussing any achievements or links to veterinary medicine. It is important to be flexible with your approach in the context of strict time limits found in MMI stations.

Question 2
What are some features of a good leader?

"A leader needs to be many things. They need to be motivational, organised and able to delegate appropriately. However in my opinion the best leaders are those who foster an environment that allows team members to feel comfortable to voice opinions and raise concerns. By doing so, the leader invites criticism in a safe environment so that conflicts or problems within any particular group or project can be addressed quickly.

An example of great leadership I have observed is the coach of my netball team. She is firm in her expectations yet when issues have arisen, such as episodes of bullying, she listens non-judgmentally to team members which enables other issues to come to light. I have tried to mimic this in my own leadership roles. For example, last year I was elected Head Girl at my school and made the effort during speeches to let the other students know that I was available to talk to them if they were facing difficulties. I hope to carry forward that approachability and ability to listen in future leadership scenarios as a vet."

Feedback
This is an excellent answer. The student gives a handful of qualities seen in good leaders, but expands on one particular element (approachability) in detail.
This answer shows reflection on a good leader from an extracurricular activity, but then demonstrates how the candidate has put what they have learnt into action in their own life.

Question 3
Practice MMI station
Station brief
What attributes do you have that will make you a good vet?

A good answer may include:
- Identification of multiple key qualities essential for veterinarians
- Acknowledgment that both 'hard' and 'soft' skills are important
- Reflection on work experience, giving an example of a situation where key skills were demonstrated by the professionals at work
- Demonstration of key skills being developed by the candidate through extracurricular activities

A poor answer may include:
- Overemphasis on academic attributes and knowledge - remember that the purpose of vet school is to teach you the medical knowledge needed to become a vet! While academic aptitude is important, in-depth medical knowledge is not required of an applicant.
- Superficial descriptions rather than deep reflection on one's own abilities and skills.

Question 5
Practice MMI station
Station brief
This station will focus on exploring your personal qualities and how these make you suitable to become a vet.

As a vet you will have to break bad news and deal with situations where things go wrong. How will you cope with this emotionally?

A good answer may:
- Understand the importance of relating to a client when breaking bad news. We need to show empathy to avoid being overly cold or clinical.
- A good candidate will also avoid being overly emotional. There is a balance between being too corporate and too sentimental. Healthcare professionals need to keep an emotional distance in order to think properly and behave appropriately.
- Reference any work experience or volunteering. Reflection on observations of difficult situations or describing how a candidate has developed their own communication skills would strengthen an answer.

A poor answer may:
- Admit that this is an area where the candidate would struggle. A surprising number of candidates respond to this question by saying they are emotional and will find breaking bad news too challenging.
- Being apathetic. Some candidates say they would approach difficult situations by being fully unemotional and detached, treating the patient as a scientific case.

Anatomy

Expert's Advice
Although some interviews will assess you on basic anatomy knowledge, understanding of anatomy teaching is not a topic that needs to be brought up at every vet school interview. Only mention it if this is an area you are particularly interested in, or if the vet school you are applying to has an interesting approach to teaching.

Question 1
Do you think you will find cadaveric dissection useful?

"To be honest, I am scared of blood and so feel a bit nervous about having to see dead animals but I will try my best to overcome my fears. I also don't think that working with cadavers will be useful as vets operate on living patients and not ones that have already died."

Applying to Veterinary Medicine

Feedback
This is a poor answer. The student fails to appreciate the unique learning experience that dissection could provide. This leaves a negative and uninterested impression on the interviewer.

"Yes of course! I am a visual learner and find that reinforcing something I read in a textbook into a real-life example will enable me to consolidate information better. I also feel it provides a far better reflection of the complexity of the specimen body than drawn-diagrams do, as they represent an accurate representation of anatomical knowledge."

Feedback
This student is enthusiastic and shows the interviewer they have reflected on dissection and can see benefits for their learning. The answer is positive and focuses on the strengths of dissection.

Question 2
Practice MMI station
Station brief
Please look at the following image and answer the following questions:

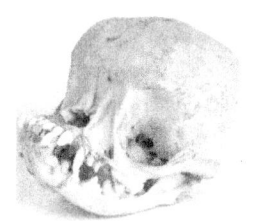

1. What is the structure in the photo?
2. Why do you think that it is this structure?
3. Can you guess what breed this structure is from?
4. Why do you think this?
5. How might this structure cause health problems compared to a 'normal' structure of this?

Answer
1. The structure in the photo is a skull from a dog.
2. The teeth look like from a carnivorous animal, eyes on the front of the head suggest this animal is a predator species (for dogs this is from their distant relatives the wolf).
3. This is a skull from a pug, although you may guess it is from another brachycephalic breed.

4. This skull looks very squashed up with a classic appearance of that belonging to a brachycephalic breed. The eye sockets are also wide and large which correlates to the 'pop eyed' appearance of pugs. Also note how the nose is completely squashed up along the top of the maxilla.
5. The design of the pug unfortunately predisposes it to many health conditions; you may mention that because all of the skull features are there but squashed up this often makes the breed likely to suffer from BOAS (brachycephalic obstructive airway syndrome). The eye sockets are wide but shallow which also means the eyeball does not sit well within the orbit, therefore often pugs can suffer from traumatic problems relating to their eyes due to the way they are sat in the skull. You may even mention the teeth and how all the teeth are squashed up too, and mention how this can relate to dental problems which pugs are prone to.

In a good answer, the candidate would:
- Correctly identify structure and state what breed it is from
- Realise the potential health problems, just from looking at the structure and using initiative to explain how the way the skull is adapted can cause problems.
- Continually explain their thought process, to help them reach their decisions.

In a poor answer, the candidate might:
- Offer superficial detail and fail to go into depth - E.g. They only say they see a skull but cannot explain why they think that.
- Fail to attempt a guess at potential health problems even if prompted with phrases - E.g. They may ask if this looks like a normal dog skull.
- Be unable to offer justification for why they think the structure is a particular part - In this case, a good candidate should relate the anatomy to BOAS. For example, just saying that a skull has dental crowding is not enough - they need to say why this anatomical change has occurred.

Expert's Advice
Every time you say a statement or make a point ask yourself "why?" This will help you develop your answer and it is what the interviewer is looking for.

Veterinary Ethics

Question 1
Practice MMI station
Station brief
You are a new graduate vet in a small, privately owned practice who is on call out of hours. You receive a call from an owner that is not registered with the practice to say their pet has been hit by a car. However, they explain to you that they have severe cost restrictions and are likely to struggle to pay for any treatment.
Discuss the different factors involved in this scenario and what you might do.

A good answer may include:
- Thinking about the different **stakeholders** involved. Whilst your first instinct may be to think of an animal who is likely suffering (and this is certainly important), what about how the owner is feeling about this situation? What about the owner of your practice, who relies on its income for their livelihood? And crucially what about you? How do you think you would feel in this situation if it happened in real life?

- Knowing your **legal responsibilities**. The RCVS code of conduct says that we have a legal obligation to provide first aid in cases like this, but this can mean different things to different people. At the very least we should be offering pain relief to make this animal comfortable, or if we do not feel this is possible then suggesting euthanasia if there is no other option.

- **Communication** is vital in situations such as this. Remaining calm and explaining clearly to the owners what you can and can't do in advance ensures realistic expectations. This is a highly stressful situation for both you and the owners and things could easily become heated if communication breaks down.

A poor answer may include:
- Being **judgemental**. As a vet you are likely to interact with all sorts of people from all sorts of backgrounds. It can be easy to think 'these people shouldn't have got a dog if they couldn't afford to care for it'. This may be true, but it is not our job to make such judgements, we must do what is best for the animal whenever this occurs.

- **Rushing** into things. Emergency situations can be very nerve-wracking, and it can be easy to make decisions quickly. We need to carry out a detailed assessment of the animal in front of us to work out what, if anything, can be done. Otherwise, we may actually end up costing our practice more money than we need to.

- Creating **unrealistic expectations**. Given the lack of finances in this case, there will be lots of scenarios where we are unable to cure the animal involved. However, as long as we can keep the animal comfortable overnight, it may be that the owners can source funds from elsewhere or we can refer them to a charity practice for further treatment.

Teaching Style

Question 1
Why do you want to study a strand/spiral learning course?

"I assume that strand or spiral learning will provide a small amount of learning that is only necessary for that year which will really help me. I sometimes struggle to concentrate when given too much information to revise so I think I will be more suited to a building on learning approach."

<u>Feedback</u>
This answer is too negative. The candidate places too much emphasis on why this learning would not suit them rather than why it will suit their learning style. This may lead the interviewer to question if the student would struggle to cope with the demands of the course.

"I find integration and applying work extremely rewarding as I feel that I am better suited to learn by understanding how what I have learnt applies to clinical practice. This is because I find it much more engaging and interactive compared to learning a large scale of information all at once"

<u>Feedback</u>
This answer uses the same key points but is framed more positively. The student focuses on the aspects of strand learning where they would thrive. This comes across as more positive and optimistic than the previous answer, and as a result the student appears enthusiastic and self-motivated.

Expert's Advice
As with other types of questions, try and use examples from previous studies to provide evidence for your main points. For example, reflecting on a school group project where you performed well and drawing comparisons to a strand learning session will help convince the admissions panel you are well suited to their curriculum.

Question 2
Why do you think the course at this vet school suits you?

"After reading your prospectus, I read up more about how rotations work in the final years of vet school. I really feel this will benefit me as I like to work in a team. I wasn't sure how I would deal with being independent in a clinical setting so decided to apply for a rotation based course as it seems like a good way to gain more confidence."

Applying to Veterinary Medicine

Feedback
This is a poor answer. The student comes across as unsure and uncommitted to the vet school. There is little reflection on their own skills or learning style, and this does little to convince the interviewer that they would be a good fit for their vet school.

"I really like how the course here prides itself on team based learning in a clinical setting, which means that I will benefit from being a leader and independent studies but also gain the benefits of natural teamworking skills. This will enable me to gain a variety of skills including engaging in peer-learning problem solving seen in clinical practice. I tend to prefer independent study at school and I am looking forward to trying out new ways seen and valued specifically in practice to be able to become the best vet possible."

Feedback
This is a better answer. The student has clearly researched the course and comes across as excited and enthusiastic. They also demonstrate a degree of reflection through the recognition of how an integrated learning style will enable the development of relevant skills needed to work in a team.

VETERINARY LIVE MMI CIRCUIT

- ✓ Written by real MMI examiners, and trusted by schools
- ✓ Perform 10 live MMI stations yourself, completing a full circuit, and then pair up to observe an additional 10 stations!
- ✓ Experience a wide range of stations, covering role plays, veterinary ethics, hot topics, work experience, and more

Book Your Place Today!

Find out more at https://www.medicmind.co.uk/vet-school-mmi-circuit/ or scan the QR code below

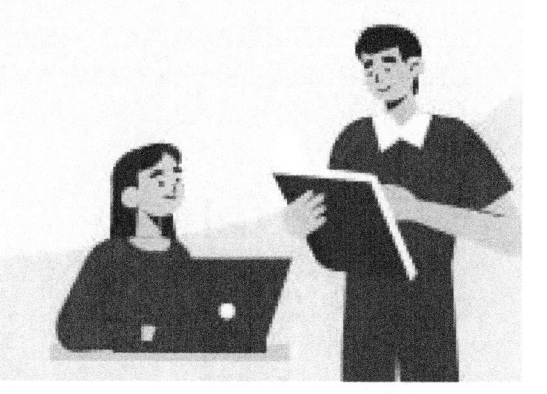

VETERINARY INTERVIEW ONLINE COURSE

- ✓ 100+ tutorials, and 100+ MMI stations, designed by our Dentistry interview experts

- ✓ Learn how to answer questions on motivation for Dentistry, personal skills, work experience, hot topics, and more

- ✓ A range of packages available, including a live day of teaching and 1:1 tutoring

Buy Now!

Find out more at https://www.medicmind.co.uk/veterinary-medicine-interview-course/ or scan the QR code below

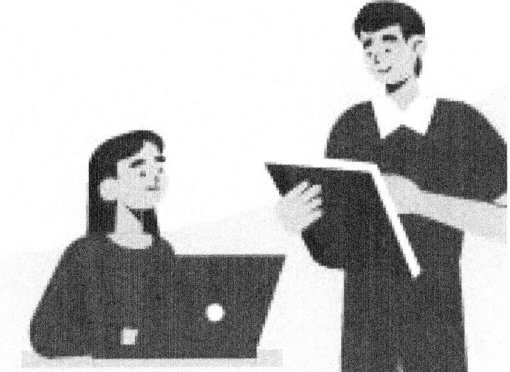

1:1 VET INTERVIEW TUTORING

✓ Delivered by current Dentistry students, who excelled in the interview themselves

✓ A personalised 1:1 approach, tailored to your unique needs

✓ An overall 93.4% success rate, with students improving their performance by an average of 57.3%

Book your FREE consultation now

For more information, visit https://www.medicmind.co.uk/vet-interview-tutors/ or scan the QR code below

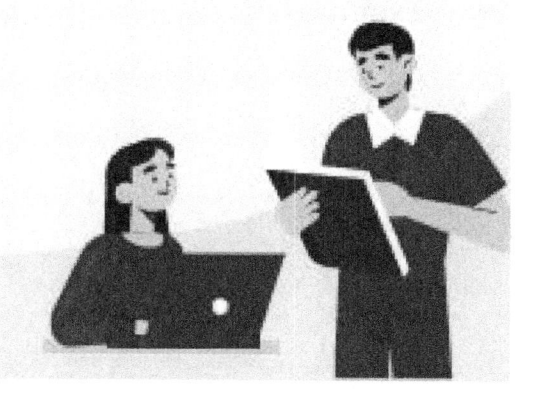

Printed in Great Britain
by Amazon